Brain Death

Brain Death

Editor

Eelco F. M. Wijdicks, M.D., Ph.D., F.A.C.P.

Professor of Neurology, Mayo Medical School
Medical Director, Neurology-Neurosurgery Intensive Care Unit
Consultant, Department of Neurology
Mayo Clinic
Rochester, Minnesota

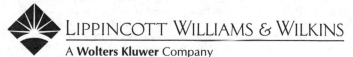

LIPPINCOTT WILLIAMS & WILKINS
A **Wolters Kluwer** Company
Philadelphia · Baltimore · New York · London
Buenos Aires · Hong Kong · Sydney · Tokyo

Acquisitions Editor: Anne Sydor
Developmental Editor: Denise Martin
Production Editor: Frank Aversa
Manufacturing Manager: Ben Rivera
Cover Designer: Mark Lerner
Compositor: Maryland Composition
Printer: Maple Press

© 2001 by **LIPPINCOTT WILLIAMS & WILKINS**
530 Walnut Street
Philadelphia, PA 19106 USA
LWW.com

Library of Congress Cataloging-in-Publication Data

Brain death : a clinical guide / edited by Eelco F. M. Wijdicks.
    p. ; cm.
  Includes bibliographical references and index.
  ISBN 0-7817-3020-1
    1. Brain death. I. Wijdicks, Eelco F. M., 1954-
  [DNLM: 1. Brain Death. W 820 B8118 2001]
  QP87 .B73 2001
  616.07'8—dc21

                               00-065523

10 9 8 7 6 5 4 3 2 1

To all who faced the worst loss but gained by giving life to others

Contents

Contributing Authors

Stephen Ashwal, M.D.   *Professor of Pediatrics and Neurology; Chief, Division of Pediatric Neurology, Loma Linda University School of Medicine, Loma Linda, California*

John L. D. Atkinson, M.D., F.A.C.S.   *Associate Professor of Neurosurgery, Mayo Medical School; Consultant, Department of Neurologic Surgery, Mayo Clinic, Rochester, Minnesota*

H. Richard Beresford, M.D.   *Adjunct Professor of Law, Myron Taylor Hall, Cornell University Law School; Professor of Neurology, University of Rochester School of Medicine, Ithaca, New York*

James L. Bernat, M.D.   *Professor of Medicine (Neurology); Associate Chief, Neurology Section, Dartmouth-Hitchcock Medical Center, Lebanon, New Hampshire*

Michael N. Diringer, M.D.   *Associate Professor of Neurology, Neurosurgery, and Anesthesiology; Director, Neurology/Neurosurgery Intensive Care Unit, Washington University School of Medicine, St. Louis, Misssouri*

Steve F. Emery, B.A., C.P.T.C.   *Procurement Transplant Coordinator, LifeSource, Upper Midwest OPO, Inc., Rochester, Minnesota*

Christine M. Gallagher, M.A.R.   *Religious Outreach Consultant, Grand Junction, Colorado*

Jan E. Leestma, M.D. M.M.   *Neuropathologist, The Chicago Institute of Neurosurgery and Neuroresearch, Columbus Hospital, Chicago, Illinois*

Kerri M. Robertson, M.D.   *Associate Clinical Professor of Anesthesiology, Department of Anesthesiology, Duke University Medical Center, Durham, North Carolina*

Eelco F. M. Wijdicks, M.D., Ph.D., F.A.C.P.   *Professor of Neurology, Mayo Medical School; Medical Director, Neurology-Neurosurgery Intensive Care Unit; Consultant, Department of Neurology, Mayo Clinic, Rochester, Minnesota*

Foreword

Brain death is an artifact of nature resulting from the capacity of medical technology to prolong and distort the process of dying. For centuries, death was signalled by the loss of breathing, but in the early nineteenth century the invention of the stethoscope switched attention to the beating heart as the essential sign of life. An immediate consequence of the arrest of either respiration or circulation is death of the brain. But when it is the brain that dies first and causes failure of respiration, a ventilator can now substitute this lost function and the heart can then continue to beat for many days. Ventilating in these circumstances deprives patients of death with dignity, prolongs the distress of families and friends, and is an inappropriate use of intensive care resources. It was to deal in practical terms with this iatrogenic dilemma that the Harvard Committee proposed criteria for the diagnosis of brain death. More than 30 years later, it is timely to review, as this volume carefully does, how thinking and practice have developed in this sensitive area of medicine.

Although the motivation for reliably diagnosing brain death was to minimize futile interventions on patients already dead, it was soon clear that its recognition afforded an opportunity for increasing the provision of organs for transplantation. Indeed this is tacitly acknowledged in the dedication of this book. It was this aspect of brain death that immediately caught the interest and imagination of the media and the public.

Reports of premature diagnosis of brain death, allegedly to facilitate organ donation, hit the press in several countries and there were soon fictional accounts in books and films of medical conspiracies to secure organs via brain death. In fact it is still only a minority of brain dead patients who become donors.

Scientific arguments about brain death *per se* have mostly been about the reliability of clinical criteria and the relevance of confirmatory laboratory tests. It is interesting that so many countries now accept the early suggestion that rigorous but simple tests are reliable (but only if all of them are always carried out), and also recognize that every confirmatory test has some limitations. As the public has come to appreciate and welcome the benefits of organ transplantation, confidence in the diagnosis of brain death has grown, and the public seems to have had little difficulty in coming to terms with the concept of brain death. At the bedside most people already know that their loved one has "gone."

Lawyers too have embraced the concept; in many countries they have legislated that when neurological criteria are met by current medical standards, a person may be declared dead. However, in Denmark and Germany it was only when laws were proposed to acknowledge what had already become accepted medical practice that a sometimes violent public debate was provoked. After much anguish, the original legal proposals were eventually accepted and the dust settled—but not until 1990 and 1997, respectively. In contrast to this, lawyers in Britain declared in 1976, when the

ix

Royal College guidelines were published, that no new law was needed—a person was dead when a physician said so, and how the physician did this was up to the medical profession. But the nationally accepted guidelines ensured more rigorous criteria than were usual for declaring "normal" somatic death, when mistakes are sometimes made and provide newspapers with stories.

Philosophers are another matter. Although most major religions have accepted brain death and approve organ transplants, some academic philosophers continue to debate the incoherence of current concepts. Are the brain dead really dead yet, they ask; and if so, is it not logical to include among the brain dead those who are in a vegetative state? In any event, why is it so important to declare a person dead before discontinuing futile treatment or taking organs? Some philosophers seem concerned that the pragmatism of physicians and the public has led too readily to the acceptance of brain death and would like to re-ignite controversy. The conclusion of a Yale lawyer, reviewing a conference proceeding on this topic, is that the U.S. needs another such divisive issue the way it needs a second hurricane Andrew. From the other side of the Atlantic I say "Amen to that."

Bryan Jennett, C.B.E., M.D., F.R.C.S.

Foreword

Since ancient times, death was believed to occur at the moment when all vital signs ceased permanently. In biological terms, it coincided with a change in animate parts of the body to inanimate. This definition satisfied religious as well as civil authorities. For those who assumed the existence of a deity as an ultimate reality, there was also a departure of the soul as well as the mind and corporal life.

For scientists and physicians whose hypotheses and theories are presumably based on verifiable observations, death in the past was also assumed to coincide with the permanent arrest of all bodily functions. And, since the mind was believed to be expressive of brain functions, the cessation of its activity was taken for granted as part of the physical effects. The status of the soul was ignored in such formulations.

In more recent times, as neuroscientists and neurologists have had the opportunity to study individuals bereft of all psychic or mental activity, they became aware of the futility of existence for such people. These individuals were unable to satisfy their "inner needs;" nor were they able to care for themselves, to procreate, or to participate in and contribute to society. Self-consciousness, emotions, memories, and identity were all effaced. For all practical purposes, the very attributes and qualities that set man apart from all other living creatures had vanished.

Was not such a person essentially dead as far as meaningful life is considered, even though his heart and circulation and other organs continued to function? That was the question that my colleagues and I asked when the "Harvard Criteria" were being enunciated.

The idea of brain death being the ultimate reality of life's end was assuredly not original with the Harvard Committee. The concept had been entertained by countless scholars. Moreover, our ideas were influenced in part by the electroencephalographic findings (EEG silence) of our colleague, Robert Schwab, and the neuropathologic findings of pannecrosis of the brain by E. P. Richardson. Again, such physiologic and pathologic findings were already known to others. Unique to the Harvard Group was the fact that Harry Beecher, a professor of anesthesiology at the Massachusetts General Hospital, had called together a neurologist, a neurosurgeon, a professor of ethics, and medical administrators of diverse academic interests to ponder the subject of brain death.

It fell upon me to draw up a set of simple, practical, and inviolable neurophysiological criteria of brain death. A permanent state of "complete unreceptivity and complete unresponsivity" was proposed. By "complete unreceptivity" was meant all stimulus effects (whether excitatory, reflexive, cognitive, or other functions) on the organism. By "complete unresponsivity" was meant all responses, whether brainstem, spinal, or cerebral in origin, including respiration. An isoelectric EEG after 24 hours and another clinical evaluation then or later were advised in order to satisfy the criterion of permanence of the state and to exclude transient disorders such as drug intoxications, concussion, and so on.

Dr. William Sweet and Dr. Beecher approved of these criteria, and they played active roles in presenting these criteria to the medical and neurological professions and to civil societies.

It is gratifying to observe that the concept of brain death has been widely accepted by the U.S.A. and elsewhere; and that it has not been abnegated by problems related to "the vegetative state" and "organ donation." This subject has attracted an enormous number of medical articles in recent years, which are thoughtfully reviewed by Dr. Eelco Wijdicks and his contributors.

Raymond D. Adams, M.D.

Preface

Consciousness, perception, emotion, memory, learning, language, personality insights, and things we do every day all originate in the brain. It is startling to be reminded that it took many thousands of years to link the brain to the soul and mind. I need hardly remind this readership of the cardiocentric view in antiquity. The unimportance of the brain can be inferred from the Egyptian embalmers who extracted organs through small openings and removed the brain via trephining the orbit or through puncture of the ethmoid bone. The brain was discarded, unlike other viscera which were buried with the dead. The Egyptians did not know what the brain was for; and as far as they were concerned, intellectual activity took place in the heart. The heart was kept in place, awaiting judgment by Anubis (god of the dead), who would weigh it against a feather (heavy from vice or light when without sin).

The hippocratic physicians can be credited with linking the brain to the mind. It is difficult to say how critical intelligence propagated itself over the years; but Herophilus of Chalcedon (circa 300 B.C.), after human dissections, emphasized that the brain transmitted motor impulses from the soul to the extremities through nerves. There was fierce opposition by Aristotle, who maintained the central position of the heart. The embryo developing within eggs had the heart beating as the first sign of life; and thus, Aristotle argued its physiologic primacy. He theorized that the "naturally cold" brain served as a refrigerator to cool the blood's heat and to adjust the organism as a whole.

Galen discovered that perception and cognition were affected by brain injury and delineated the cranial nerves; and Willis, to name a few leading scientists, further differentiated the cerebral functions and championed neuroanatomy, culminating in the work *Cerebri Anatome*.

Little do we know of the unimaginable complexity of the workings of three billion neurons that make up the human brain, but we know when its function ceases. When the brain dies, human life is taken; and it is the end of everything here. Although this may be obvious to the point of a platitude, a few theorists and cultures are not at peace with it. Some intellectuals believe brain death is not a fixed absolute and continue to debate the concept.

I began this book with the proposition that brain death means not only a nonsapient state but death, and this book displays a hard core of common sense in setting it out. Brain death has undeniable fascination. But, this monograph takes no part in sensationalism and quasi-certainties but brings to the fore a few of the polarities in analysis of the subject matter.

Death by neurologic criteria has become an accepted method of diagnosis of clinical death; however, the complexities of the clinical diagnosis and evaluation of potential pitfalls in brain death remain substantial. *Brain Death* covers a great deal of ground but is framed around the most pertinent components of clinical evaluation of patients. In addition, it focuses on religious, legal, ethical, and philosophical aspects. The authors, from all involved specialties, are practicing experts in the field and have provided their best work. I have retained some overlap to allow the contributors to develop their arguments. New material, after thorough research of hidden resources and interviews, has been included. This book not only helps readers to review knowledge on brain death, it essentially provides a clinically useful text for practitioners seeing patients with acute catastrophic neurologic disorders evolving to brain death. I hope it will appeal to neurologists, neuro-intensivists, neurosurgeons, anesthesiologists, trauma surgeons, neuroscience and intensive care nursing staff, transplantation surgeons, and organ procurement organizations.

Eelco F. M. Wijdicks, M.D., Ph.D.

Acknowledgments

The topic of brain death has never been simple to me. Attempting a fresh reading of a potentially desiccated topic has been rewarding thanks to many resources. I offer thanks to many librarians who helped in finding historical sources and photographs—particularly Andy Lucas of the Mayo Historical Unit. Nicole Perrault translated the "*Le Coma Dépassé*" article and related manuscripts that offered a more convincing picture of the earlier years of evolution of the criteria of brain death. I am particularly grateful for the illuminating correspondence with Professor Takeshita, who took me through the cultural landscape of Japan and its historical "minefields." I greatly welcomed the commentaries of earlier pioneers, Professor Bryan Jennett and Professor Raymond Adams, which contain a masterful assemblage of insights into the U.K. and U.S. positions during the development of clinical criteria.

The secretarial help (Donna Asleson and many others) at the Mayo Medical Center has been superb. My secretary, Tammy Drees, gave energy and time beyond the call of duty. I thank the Section of Scientific Publications—specifically, Werner Heidel for editing, and Sharon Wadleigh for organization and formatting. My wife, Barbara-Jane, and children, Coen and Marilou, endured the vacant stare of a husband and father immersed in a complex subject, but they were a beacon of love and understanding.

I also thank Anne Sydor, Acquisitions Editor, and Denise Martin, Developmental Editor, of Lippincott Williams & Wilkins for the timely production of this book.

Eelco F. M. Wijdicks, M.D., Ph.D.

INTRODUCTION

The Landmark *"Le Coma Dépassé"*

Eelco F. M. Wijdicks

Department of Neurology, Mayo Clinic, Rochester, Minnesota

Un tel coma est à la fois une révélation et une rançon de la maîtrise acquise en matière de réanimation neuro-respiratoire.—P. Mollaret and M. Goulon (1)

The article by Mollaret and Goulon was an extension of earlier anecdotal observations by others of comatose patients with absent electroencephalographic recordings, absent intracranial flow, or total brain necrosis at autopsy. The article, in *Revue Neurologique* in 1959, is a signature piece in the development of clinical criteria of death by neurologic standards (1) (Fig. 1). The authors presented 23 cases from the Claude Bernard Hospital in Paris with a new type of coma they called *"le coma dépassé"*— that is, coma associated with complete lack of cognitive and vegetative functions which went well beyond the deepest comas so far described. It is best translated as "irreversible or irretrievable coma" (M. Goulon, personal communication).

Although both authors (Figs. 2 and 3) used the term in their hospital service for several years before publication, they were dissatisfied with it. In fact, they encouraged the reader to propose a better term (1). Later, more nebulous terms were suggested by others, such as "deanimation encephalopathy," "supracoma," "acute necrotic anencephalie" (2), and "aperceptivity areactive apathic and atonic syndrome" (3). Interestingly, "irreversible coma" became the title of the Harvard Report in 1968, although the committee members responsible for the report were not aware of this document (R. Adams, personal communication).

As pointed out in the citation at the beginning of this introduction, the authors believed that "such a coma was not only a revelation but also a price one has to pay from the skills acquired in resuscitation."

Professors Mollaret and Goulon argued that this "revelation" was due to several technologic developments that guaranteed "survival." These advances were intubation and mechanical ventilation, control of circulation using "intravenous noradrenaline," and management of electrolyte disturbances.

The authors correctly asked the most critical ethical questions. Do we have the right to stop resuscitation using criteria that pretend to know the boundary of life and death? Does life support have to be maintained as long as the heart beats and perfuses vital organs? How about the religious position? (Pope Pius XII apparently felt that questions about the moment of death were not a matter for the church to resolve. The authors cite the solemn words of the pope himself in *Nouvelles de Chrétienté* 1957;150: 5–10.) Professor Goulon felt it was a disturbing condition for an observer and led

REVUE NEUROLOGIQUE

MÉMOIRES ORIGINAUX

LE COMA DÉPASSÉ
(MEMOIRE PRÉLIMINAIRE)

PAR MM.

P. MOLLARET et M. GOULON

Après quatre années de réflexion, nous croyons venu le moment d'ajouter un chapitre nouveau au domaine traditionnel des comas.

Précisons de suite que ce problème du coma dépassé a été mis, l'année dernière, au programme de la prochaine Journée de Réanimation de l'Hôpital Claude-Bernard du 7 octobre 1959, en vue d'une mise au point intégrale.

La présente communication, qui n'a ainsi qu'une valeur préliminaire, peut être offerte, peut-être, en hommage à la XXIIIe Réunion Neurologique Internationale, qui a accepté de tenir une de ses séances dans le Centre de Réanimation où fut élaboré ce travail. Précisons également que le coma dépassé a déjà conquis droit de cité dans l'important volume qui vient de paraître de H. Fischgold et P. Mathis (*Obnubilations, comas et stupeurs*, Masson édit., Paris, 1959, p. 5 et pp. 51-52) ; nous remercions ces auteurs d'être venus se faire présenter les premiers malades et d'avoir donné place à quelques-uns de nos documents.

FIG. 1. Original cover page of the article "*Le Coma Dépassé.*" (From Mollaret P, Goulon M. *Le coma dépassé. Rev Neurol* 1959;101:3–15, with permission of Masson Editeur.)

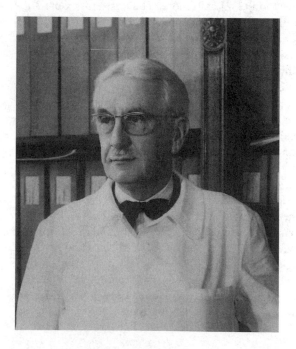

FIG. 2. Professor P. Mollaret. (Kindly provided by Professor Goulon.)

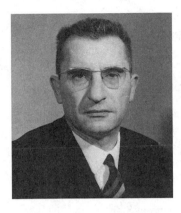

FIG. 3. Professor M. Goulon. (Kindly provided by Professor Goulon.)

him to question "where the patient's soul dwelled" (M. Goulon, personal communication).

In addition to their foresight of future ethical quandaries, they presented a well-documented description of what is now called "brain death." The following aspects were discussed in their paper: circumstances, neurologic examination, results of electroencephalography, and the consequences of brain death on functioning of other organs that were suddenly independent of control of the brain but were artificially maintained. A variety of major injuries to the brain were seen, including trauma, subarachnoid hemorrhage, meningitis, cerebral venous thrombosis, massive stroke, and brain death after craniotomy for posterior fossa tumor.

In retrospect, the paper's details of the neurologic examination are striking. *Coma dépassé* was said to be characterized by immobility of the eyeballs in a neutral position, mydriasis, absent light reflex, absent blinking with stimuli, absence of swallowing reflexcs, "drooping of the jaw," absence of motor responses to any stimuli, muscle hypotonia, tendon areflexia, equivocal plantar reflexes, "retention of idiomuscular contraction with muscle edema," absence of "medullary automatism" and sphincter incontinence, absence of spontaneous respiration after discontinuation of ventilation, immediate cardiovascular collapse as soon as the noradrenaline infusion is stopped, and a disturbance of thermoregulation–hypothermia or hyperthermia–depending on the environmental temperature.

The electroencephalogram (EEG) is flat without any noticeable reactivity, and it remains so until cardiac arrest. The authors here warn the reader, very appropriately, that a flat EEG by itself does not permit a diagnosis of *coma dépassé*. They cite personal observations, in which a flattening of the EEG can be followed by resumption of normal electrical cerebral activity, but details about the cause in such cases are not provided.

Mollaret and Goulon noted cases in which mechanical ventilation was controlled in the first days, only to deteriorate later, and they documented oxygen desaturation, acute hypercapnia, and combined respiratory and metabolic acidosis. These changes were attributed to alveoli-capillary changes from "edema and blood stasis." Polyuria was present in most cases, and intramuscular injection of "d'hormone posthypophysaire" resulted in reduced diuresis and concentration of urine. Hyperglycemia and glycosuria were observed, but there was a normal response to insulin. Hypernatremia was found in one case, which, according to the authors, attested to inadequate fluid balance. The heart rate slowed to 40 to 60 beats per minute and was not changed by pressure on the eyeballs or carotid sinus or by intravenous injection of atropine. This condition ended ultimately with cardiac arrest (2).

When we take a close look at this manuscript, it is a landmark for a number of reasons. For one thing, it distinguished *coma dépassé* from other types of comatose states. For another, it brought us a comprehensive clinical and EEG description together with the observations of diabetes insipidus, vascular collapse, and neurogenic pulmonary edema, all major derangements facing modern neurointensivists and neurosurgeons. It is a fine example of academic medicine. It took more than 15 years before it became known in the United Kingdom and the United States.

REFERENCES

1. Mollaret P, Goulon M. *Le coma dépassé. Rev Neurol* 1959;101:3–15.
2. Goulon M, Nouailhat F, Babinet P. Irreversible coma [French]. *Ann Med Interne (Paris)* 1971; 122:479–486.
3. Jouvet M. Coma and other disorders of consciousness. In: Vinken PJ, Bruyn GW, eds. *Handbook of clinical neurology. Vol. 3: disorders of higher nervous activity.* Amsterdam: North-Holland Publishing Company, 1969:62–79.

1

Brain Death in Historical Perspective

Michael N. Diringer[*] and Eelco F. M. Wijdicks[†]

*Department of Neurology, Neurosurgery and Anesthesiology, Washington University,
St. Louis, Missouri, and †Department of Neurology, Mayo Clinic, Rochester, Minnesota.*

Death took on a different meaning after Bjorn Ibsen invented the mechanical ventilator and patients with catastrophic brain injury, prone to respiratory arrest, were artificially supported in hospitals throughout the world. This unprecedented, and certainly drastic, intervention in these patients forced the emergence of a new neurologic
state. In this comatose state, brain function came to an end. The view that has pre-
vailed in civilized nations since the first comprehensive description by Mollaret and
Goulon is that we are dead when our brains are dead. In a sense, without our brain we
have permanently lost not only our personhood, identity, and soul but also its essential role in controlling systemic function and vital organs. This fundamental position
has not been questioned although differences of emphasis persist today.

Our ability to determine death with certainty continues to be questioned by scholars and social scientists; however, little, if any, controversy has persisted among
physicians (1,2). Philosophy, theology, technology, ethics, law, politics, and eco-
nomics have all influenced the definition of death. Robert Joynt wrote when remi-
niscing on the Ad Hoc Harvard Committee special communication in 1984: "the effect of the report touched almost all branches of medicine, opened new areas of law,
and posed new and different problems for theologist and ethicist. . . . It has made
physicians into lawyers, lawyers into physicians, and both into philosophers" (3).

According to Pernick, physicians may use different criteria and diagnostic tools for
defining death, but the essential questions remain the same (4). In determining death,
society has to address two questions: First, does the essence of life reside in a single
organ or is it represented throughout all organs, and second, how can we avoid, with
maximum certainty, the inaccurate diagnosis of death?

The development of neurological criteria for death began with a new definition of
death: loss of brain function. Beecher said that "we should, first, abandon the ancient
sign of death—the cessation of the heartbeat" (5). Once the definition was established, criteria had to be developed.

Several operational approaches can be used to develop criteria. One is to delineate
a state of cerebral unresponsiveness from which survival of bodily function has never
been seen. Another is to define a state that will reliably predict widespread severe
brain necrosis. A third is to define death based on indirect physiological measures of
brain function, e.g., demonstrating an isoelectric electroencephalogram (EEG) or absent cerebral blood flow.

This chapter traces the evolution of neurological criteria used for establishing
death. What has come about is recognition of reliable tests utilized through the world.

DEVELOPING NEUROLOGIC CRITERIA FOR DEATH

The initial attempt to define death based on neurological criteria is often attributed to the 1968 Harvard Criteria (6). But the first steps toward using loss of cerebral function to define death actually began several years earlier.

Lofstedt and von Reis (7) reported in 1956, six mechanically ventilated patients with absent reflexes, apnea, hypotension, hypothermia, and polyuria. Cerebral blood flow, determined by angiography, was absent. Death was declared following cardiac arrest, which occurred in 2 to 26 days. Cerebral necrosis was present at autopsy in all cases. In 1959, Wertheimer, Jouvet, and Descotes were among the first to propose criteria for these comatose states ("A propos du diagnostic de la mort système nerveux . . . "). This manuscript largely focused, as many before, on the significance of the isoelectric electroencephalogram, but also documented shutting off the ventilator to produce "prolonged apnea" in order to stimulate the respiratory centers with increasing respiratory acidosis. Absent medulla oblongata function was further confirmed with no change in pulse rate with carotid compression, ocular pressure, and intravenous injection of atropine and amphetamine (8). Both these brilliant reports, however, lacked the neurologic finesse to dissect brain death from other neurologic conditions.

Several months later in 1959, Mollaret and Goulon (9) coined the term "*le coma dépassé*" and defined death based on neurologic criteria. The paper was published in *Revue Neurologique,* a well-acknowledged journal, but was wholly unnoticed outside Europe.

In 1963 Schwab and associates (10) reported on the electroencephalogram: "EEG as an aid in determining death in the presence of cardiac activity." They pointed out that "new cardiac stimulation techniques" and mechanical ventilation often resulted in cases in which anoxia was so prolonged that "destruction to the respiratory centers and higher nervous system occurred, but where cardiac function was restored." They referred, in these unfortunate patients, to a resulting "human heart-lung preparation that may be viable for many days," as Mollaret and Goulon had done earlier, and set about using EEG as a tool for determining brain death. They proposed that the following criteria would allow the physician to indicate that the patient was dead: (a) absence of spontaneous respiration for 30 min, (b) no tendon reflexes of any type, (c) no pupillary reflexes, (d) absence of the oculocardiac reflex (eyeball pressure slowing heart rate), and (e) 30 min of isoelectric EEG.

The burgeoning field of organ transplantation unleashed a strong desire to expand the recipient pool. About the same time, the widespread use of mechanical ventilation established the need to redefine death while the heart was still beating in cases of hopeless neurologic injury. These two issues eventually united in the concept of using organs to salvage other lives. To say that brain death served to facilitate transplantation is surely not true. It is significant to know that initially there was considerable controversy about retrieving organs from patients whose cardiac function had not yet ceased. In 1966, the proceedings from a Ciba symposium on transplantation were published. Joseph Murray, a future member of the Harvard ad hoc committee and future Nobel laureate (11), described in a paper entitled "Organ Transplantation:

The Practical Possibilities," what he saw as the options for the future of organ transplantation. This was followed by a dialogue among several transplant surgeons that included discussion of potential sources of organ donors (relatives, prisoners, cadavers, and heart-beating donors without brain function). It was pointed out that related donors are not always available, the use of prisoner donors has serious ethical problems, and that the quality of organs from cadaveric donors was poor. Despite the fact that organs from heart-beating donors who had lost all brain function were considered the best option for the recipient, there was formidable resistance to this approach. Some felt that there was not sufficient "infallible evidence" to justify a legal redefinition of death. Most telling of all in this discussion, Alexandre suggested that two separate teams be involved, one working to resuscitate the patient and the other dealing with transplantation. In addition, he proposed adoption of criteria that had already been applied by his group in nine patients with severe cerebral injuries to harvest organs (11).

These criteria were basically from Mollaret and Goulon's paper (9) known to Alexandre (who was versed in French) but not to other members of the symposium. The criteria were as follows: (a) complete bilateral mydriasis, (b) complete absence of reflexes in response to pain, (c) complete absence of respiration for 5 min, (d) falling blood pressure necessitating increasing doses of vasopressors, and (e) a flat EEG for "several hours."

These criteria were by no means accepted and the responses reflected uneasiness and strong opposition. Starzl, a budding pioneer in liver transplantation, stated, "I doubt if any of the members of our transplantation team could accept a person as being dead as long as there was a heartbeat." Another transplant surgeon, Calne, noted: "Although Alexandre's criteria are medically persuasive according to traditional definitions of death, he is in fact removing kidneys from live donors. I feel that if a patient has a heartbeat he cannot be regarded as a cadaver." Calne predicted this would become a very sensitive issue. "Any modification of the means of diagnosing death to facilitate transplantation will cause the whole procedure to fall into disrepute with the rest of the profession." Only Murray expressed enthusiasm, "Those criteria are excellent." "This is the kind of formulation that we will need before we can approach the legal profession." Revillard proposed adding two additional criteria: (a) demonstrating absence of cerebral blood flow by angiography and (b) absence of a reaction to atropine, but disagreed with falling blood pressure because it may remain at 100 mm Hg for several hours.

The proposed criteria called for (a) a consultation with three physicians, one of whom should be the Hospital Chief of Service; (b) a written report of the evaluation be prepared with a copy for each signator, the hospital and the authorities; (c) proof of existence of irreversible lesions inconsistent with survival; (d) loss of all reflexes; (e) fixed dilated pupils; (f) a flat EEG or the demonstration of extensive directly observed lesion (e.g., open head wound); and (g) respiration and circulation were entirely supported ("incapable of maintaining life in the absence of artificial methods").

The conference ended without resolution of the dispute and no final recommendations were forthcoming.

In 1968 the Harvard Medical School ad hoc Committee to Examine the Definition of Brain Death (6) set out to "define irreversible coma as a new criterion for death." The committee had representatives of the Harvard University Medical School, School of Public Health, Divinity School, Graduate School, and Law School, chaired by Henry Beecher, an anesthesiologist (Fig. 1-1), and included neurologists Raymond Adams (see Foreword) and Denny-Brown and neurosurgeon Sweet. The committee chose to philosophically define death as irreversible loss of all brain function, and then proposed the criteria necessary to make that determination. The criteria were not subject to empirical confirmation; rather they were based on the collective experience of the committee members. The document, a patched collection of brief statements included definitions of brain death, a legal commentary and an address by his holiness Pope Pius XII. It was published in the *Journal of the American Medical Association (JAMA)* on August 5, 1968. The paper, a special communication, was insensitively flanked by a paper on plague and a paper on ethical guidelines for organ transplantation, and to top it off, the cover of *JAMA* showed an artistic depiction of black death (Fig. 1-2).

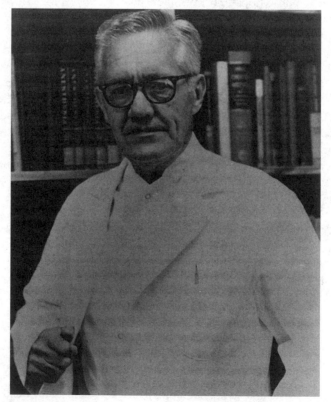

FIG. 1-1. Portrait of Henry Beecher, with permission of the Massachusetts General Hospital (Archives and Special Collections).

JAMA

VOL 205, NO 6   AUGUST 5, 1968

THE JOURNAL
of the
American Medical Association

*Continuing Education
Courses for Physicians*

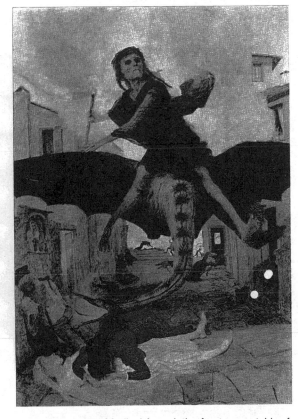

The Swiss painter, Arnold Böcklin, frequently introduced a mythological atmosphere into his work. Here "Plague," executed in 1898 during the last world pandemic, is shown as Death astride a black batwinged monster. It was that epidemic which brought plague to the western United States, whence the infection became transmitted to native wild rodents, as sylvatic plague, occasionally transmitted back to man (see p 333). The original of the painting is from the Gottfried Keller Foundation, in the Basel Art Museum, Switzerland.

FIG. 1-2. Title page of the *Journal of the American Medical Association* front cover, table of contents, and the special communication of the Harvard criteria. (From *JAMA*, vol. 205, August 5, 1968. By permission of the American Medical Association.)

The committee stated that the clinical diagnosis required unreceptivity and unresponsivity, and no movements or breathing, and absence of brainstem reflexes (Table 1-1). The term "unreceptivity" was introduced to exclude locked in syndrome that greatly concerned neurologists because it could mimic brain death. An isoelectric EEG was considered "of great confirmatory value," and its use was recommended, when available. In order to determine that the state was not reversible, all tests were

ORIGINAL CONTRIBUTIONS

SPECIAL COMMUNICATION

JUDICIAL COUNCIL

MEDICAL WRITING—NO 24

NEGATIVE RESULTS

DIAGNOSTIC PROCEDURES

THERAPEUTIC GRAND ROUNDS—NO 5

CONTINUING EDUCATION COURSES FOR PHYSICIANS

(Contents continued on reverse side)

FIG. 1-2. *Continued.*

A Definition of
Irreversible Coma

Report of the Ad Hoc Committee of the Harvard Medical School
to Examine the Definition of Brain Death

Our primary purpose is to define irreversible coma as a new criterion for death. There are two reasons why there is need for a definition: (1) Improvements in resuscitative and supportive measures have led to increased efforts to save those who are desperately injured. Sometimes these efforts have only partial success so that the result is an individual whose heart continues to beat but whose brain is irreversibly damaged. The burden is great on patients who suffer permanent loss of intellect, on their families, on the hospitals, and on those in need of hospital beds already occupied by these comatose patients. (2) Obsolete criteria for the definition of death can lead to controversy in obtaining organs for transplantation.

Irreversible coma has many causes, but *we are concerned here only with those comatose individuals who have no discernible central nervous system activity*. If the characteristics can be defined in satisfactory terms, translatable into action—and we believe this is possible—then several problems will either disappear or will become more readily soluble.

More than medical problems are present. There are moral, ethical, religious, and legal issues. Adequate definition here will prepare the way for better insight into all of these matters as well as for better law than is currently applicable.

The Ad Hoc Committee includes Henry K. Beecher, MD, chairman; Raymond D. Adams, MD; A. Clifford Barger, MD; William J. Curran, LLM, SMHyg; Derek Denny-Brown, MD; Dana L. Farnsworth, MD; Jordi Folch-Pi, MD; Everett I. Mendelsohn, PhD; John P. Merrill, MD; Joseph Murray, MD; Ralph Potter, ThD; Robert Schwab, MD; and William Sweet, MD.
Reprint requests to Massachusetts General Hospital, Boston 02114 (Dr. Henry K. Beecher).

Characteristics of Irreversible Coma

An organ, brain or other, that no longer functions and has no possibility of functioning again is for all practical purposes dead. Our first problem is to determine the characteristics of a *permanently* nonfunctioning brain.

A patient in this state appears to be in deep coma. The condition can be satisfactorily diagnosed by points 1, 2, and 3 to follow. The electroencephalogram (point 4) provides confirmatory data, and when available it should be utilized. In situations where for one reason or another electroencephalographic montioring is not available, the absence of cerebral function has to be determined by purely clinical signs, to be described, or by absence of circulation as judged by standstill of blood in the retinal vessels, or by absence of cardiac activity.

1. *Unreceptivity and Unresponsitivity.*—There is a total unawareness to externally applied stimuli and inner need and complete unresponsiveness—our definition of irreversible coma. Even the most intensely painful stimuli evoke no vocal or other response, not even a groan, withdrawal of a limb, or quickening of respiration.

2. *No Movements or Breathing.*—Observations covering a period of at least one hour by physicians is adequate to satisfy the criteria of no spontaneous muscular movements or spontaneous respiration or response to stimuli such as pain, touch, sound, or light. After the patient is on a mechanical respirator, the total absence of spontaneous breathing may be established by turning off the respirator for three minutes and observing whether there is any effort on the part of the subject to breathe

FIG. 1-2. *Continued.*

to be repeated in 24 h. While it was not necessary to determine the etiology of the coma, neurologic examination had to be performed in the absence of hypothermia or sedative drugs. Once the determination was made, the report indicated that the family should be informed, death be declared, and the respirator turned off. It was suggested that the physician in charge of the patient consult with one or more other physicians "so that the responsibility is shared over a wide range of medical opinion."

The common problem of contexts was further illustrated in the next issue of *JAMA*, which provided several contributions on transplantation, including an editorial of Appel, former president of the American Medical Association. He opened, "might not the over enthusiastic heart surgeon be tempted to declare the donor dead before

TABLE 1-1. *Harvard criteria (1968)*

Unreceptivity and unresponsivity
No movements or breathing
No reflexes
Flat electroencephalogram
All of the above four tests shall be repeated at, at least, 24 h with no change
Exclusion of hypothermia (below 90°F or 32.2°C) or central nervous system depressants

From "A definition of irreversible coma: report of the Ad Hoc Committee of the Harvard Medical School to Examine the Definition of Brain Death." *JAMA* 1968;205:337–340, with permission.

death occurred in order to have a viable heart to transplant," and followed by many questions about the ethical implications of transplantation, rousing debate (12).

The Harvard Criteria were published in 1968, one of the most turbulent years in the United States. Overwhelmed with other news, the media relegated the Harvard Criteria to the news of minor interest (*Newsweek*, August 19, 1968, published a small column on a page ironically also carrying an article about physician errors). Some influential major newspapers such as the *New York Times* did report its publication on the front page (Fig. 1-3) and gave the committee high marks, but a passage in their editorial page entitled "Redefining Death" reflected the common public confusion with the vegetative state: "As old as medicine is the question of what to do about the human vegetable . . . Sometimes these living corpses have survived for years . . . It is such cases, as well as the needs for organs to be transplanted that the Harvard faculty committee had in mind in urging that death be redefined as irreversible coma" (*New*

Harvard Panel Asks Definition of Death Be Based on Brain

By ROBERT REINHOLD

A special faculty committee at Harvard University has recommended that the definition of death be based on "brain death," even though the heart may continue to beat. The committee offered a set of guidelines for physicians to determine when such death occurs.

The 13-man panel was drawn from the university's faculties of medicine, public health, law, divinity and arts and sciences.

The panel said its action was prompted by the possibility that "obsolete criteria" for death might lead to controversy in organ transplants and in modern resuscitative methods, which can maintain heartbeat in comatose patients with irreversible brain damage.

In a report, to be published today in the Journal of the American Medical Association under the title "A Definition of Irreversible Coma," the committee urges physicians to accept new standards for determining the moment of death as a prelude to a change in the legal definition.

FIG. 1-3. Front page of the *New York Times* (August 5, 1968) announcing the Harvard Criteria for Brain Death. By permission of the New York Times Company.

York Times, August 5, 1968). In America, the startling news of new death criteria, was overshadowed by the Republican Party National Convention and show of force with Russian tanks in Czechoslovakia weeks later, and the publication did not foster a public debate.

We must recognize that the Ad Hoc Harvard Committee was primarily concerned with futility of care and finding ways to help physicians with withdrawal of support. Facilitating transplantation was not a major objective. To mention but one example, a follow-up communication by Beecher, Adams, and Sweet provided criteria for withdrawal of support in cases of the brain death syndrome (13). Organ donation as a potential consequence of this comatose state was not mentioned. The Committee wisely recommended that the decision to withdraw ventilation not be made by those physicians involved in organ or tissue transplantation.

Also in 1968, two German authors published a paper entitled "The Dissociated Brain Death" in the journal *Minnesota Medicine* (14). They applied the criteria of Schwab and argued that EEG was the "most reliable instrument because it is the only objective measure whereby brain function can be absolutely measured." The authors emphasized that it was essential to establish irreversibility and exclude confounding metabolic factors. All of the 12 patients included in the report suffered cardiac arrest within 60 h due to "the reciprocity of brain function with physiological integrity" (14).

The following year Adams and Jequier published "The Brain Death Syndrome: Hypoxemic Panencephalopathy" (15). They emphasized that the syndrome was a clinical diagnosis and should not rely on EEG. They exclaimed: "The physician that would permit such a crucial decision be made by a machine, ingenious as it might be, leaves himself (and his patient) in a highly vulnerable position."

In 1969 Beecher wrote in an editorial in the *New England Journal of Medicine* that the definition of irreversible coma proposed by the Committee was well accepted by the medical community but not in legal circles (16). He pointed out that "the committee was unanimous in its belief that an EEG was not essential to a diagnosis of irreversible coma, but it could provide valuable supporting data." A year later in a comment Beecher introduced a yet unpublished study by Silverman, Saunders and Schwartz of 1,667 individuals with flat EEG over 24 h or more without any recovering (5).

In a natural history study in 1970, Becker and colleagues reported on fifteen patients who met the Harvard Criteria and continued to receive all necessary medical support (17). They indicated that, despite "maximal" cardiovascular and respiratory support, nine of the 15 developed cardiac arrest in less than 24 h and the remainder did so by 50 h. This led them to question the need for a 24-h period of observation to provide evidence of irreversibility.

Mohandas and Chou published in 1971 the Minnesota Code of Brain Death Criteria in *Journal of Neurosurgery*, also known as the "Minnesota Criteria" (Table 1-2) (18). Major changes that were evident included definition of time of apnea (4 min of disconnection), "ruling out of metabolic factors," and shorter observation time of 12 h, however, none with validating facts. Mohandas and Chou first introduced into the literature that damage of the brainstem was a critical component of severe brain dam-

TABLE 1-2. *Minnesota criteria (1971)*

Known but irreparable intracranial lesion
Metabolic factors ruled out
No spontaneous movement
Apnea (4 min)
Absent brainstem reflexes: pupillary, corneal, ciliospinal, vestibulo-ocular, oculocephalic, gag
All findings unchanged for 12 h

From Mohandas A, Chou SN. Brain death—a clinical and pathologic study. *J Neurosurg* 1971;35:211–218, with permission.

age. They stated, "What we are attempting to define and establish, beyond reasonable doubt is the state of irreversible damage to the brainstem." "It is the point of no return." In addition, they stressed the irrelevance of EEG: "We also had instances in which there was electrical activity of the brain recorded; but pathologically, the brainstem was completely autolyzed in one case and extensively hemorrhagic in the other two cases." "If the clinical-neurophysiological criteria of brain death are met, the value of an EEG examination is extremely questionable" (18). This principle was further brought to maturity by United Kingdom neurologists, notably Pallis (19). The Conference of the Royal Colleges and Faculties of the United Kingdom published the "Diagnosis of Brain Death" (20) in 1976, and, in 1995, changed brain death into brainstem death: "The clinical criteria for the diagnosis of brain stem death . . . have been confirmed by all published sources and have therefore been adequately validated" (21) (Table 1-3). It resulted from 2 years of discussion between anesthesiologists, neurologists, neurophysiologists, and neurosurgeons in the United Kingdom. The United Kingdom's position was "if the brain stem is dead, the brain is dead, and if the brain is dead, the person is dead" (19–21). Therefore, an EEG, cerebral angiography, or other blood flow studies were not required. Detailed and meticulous as it

TABLE 1-3. *The United Kingdom code (1976)*

Patient deeply comatose
No depressant drugs
No hypothermia
No remediable metabolic or endocrine disturbance as cause
Spontaneous ventilation inadequate or absent
Muscle relaxants and depressant drugs excluded
Cause established, condition due to irremediable structural brain damage
Diagnostic tests
Pupils nonreactive to light
No corneal reflexes
Vestibulo-ocular reflexes absent
Stimulation anywhere elicits no motor responses mediated via cranial nerves
No gag or tracheal suction reflex
No respiratory movements when ventilator removed and $Paco_2$ rises above threshold (50 mm Hg)

From the Conference of Medical Royal Colleges and Faculties of the United Kingdom. Diagnosis of brain death. *BMJ* 1976;2:1187, with permission.

was, the Conference did require that the etiology of the condition be fully established and a search for factors that could potentially mimic loss of brainstem function. The presence of depressant drugs, neuromuscular blocking agents, respiratory depressants, and metabolic or endocrine disturbances was emphasized. A flexible period of observation was recommended, such that prolonged observation was needed in cases of hypoxic or ischemic injury, whereas only a few hours might be needed following severe head injury or intracerebral hemorrhage. Finally, the technique for apnea testing was refined to include preoxygenation, continued oxygen administration during apnea, administration of 5% CO_2 to raise arterial CO_2 to at least 50 mm Hg, and expert investigation in patients with advanced chronic respiratory insufficiency.

The public trust in the U.K. Code criteria was influenced in a negative way by a BBC program panorama viewed by 8 million under the following title: "Transplants—Are the Donors Really Dead?" (22). Three far-reaching arguments were put forward and echoed some of the earlier concerns raised in the United States after dissemination of the Harvard Criteria: (a) brain death criteria were not properly discussed before its publication, (b) the criteria were developed because of the need to find organs, and, more disturbing, (c) the criteria were not reliable. American physicians interviewed about the criteria in the United Kingdom claimed that, due to emphasis on the brainstem alone, their patients not infrequently recovered. The television broadcast fueled a public mistrust but a subsequent program made by physicians nominated by the Royal College which left little room for misinterpretation went a long way in restoring the public's trust. In fact, the "recovered" patients from the United States had been diagnosed by criteria judged inadequate by U.K. standards. The British position has been eloquently summarized by Pallis and Harley in the *ABC of Brain Stem Death* (23).

The only prospective attempt to develop guidelines for the declaration of death based on neurological criteria was performed by the NIH-sponsored multicenter U.S. Collaborative Study of Cerebral Death in 1977 (24). The goal was to develop operational criteria for a definition of death based on loss of neurological function. The project sought to prospectively identify neurological factors that would predict somatic death within 3 months despite continued cardiopulmonary support, and establish those factors as the neurological criteria for death.

To be enrolled a patient had to demonstrate cerebral unresponsivity and apnea. Of the 503 patients who met these criteria, 87% died based on cardiopulmonary criteria within 3 months. Only 19 of the 503 patients met the Harvard Criteria, and all 19 succumbed to cardiopulmonary death. The Harvard Criteria were 100% specific but very insensitive. Therefore a third set of criteria was applied: cerebral unresponsiveness, apnea, and one isoelectric EEG. Of the 189 patients who met these criteria, 187 died somatic death; the two who survived were cases of drug intoxication. The final recommended criteria (Table 1-4) required one examination at least 6 h after the onset of coma and apnea (unlike the 24 h required by the Harvard Criteria). The examination had to demonstrate cerebral unresponsivity, dilated pupils, absent brainstem reflexes, apnea, and an isoelectric EEG. Apnea was defined as the need for controlled ventilation for at least 15 min, that is, the patient made no effort to override the ven-

TABLE 1-4. *U.S. Collaborative Study criteria (1977)*

Basic prerequisite—completion of all appropriate therapeutic procedures
Unresponsive coma
Apnea
Absent cephalic reflexes with dilated, fixed pupils
Isoelectric EEG
Persistence of the above for 30 min to 1 h, 6 h after onset of coma and apnea
Optional confirmatory test indicating absence of cerebral circulation

From "An appraisal of the criteria of cerebral death: a summary statement. A collaborative study." *JAMA* 1977;237:982–986, with permission.

tilator but was not disconnected from it. Although it was recognized that not all brain-dead patients had dilated pupils, the requirement was included to avoid incorrect diagnosis in cases of drug intoxication. It was noted that spinal reflexes were poor indicators of loss of brain function and were present in approximately a third of the patients that died. Additional "confirmatory" tests to demonstrate absence of cerebral blood flow were recommended when an early diagnosis was desired, particularly when brainstem reflexes were unable to be tested or when sedatives had been administered. Finally the report recognized that the criteria were redundant but preferred the added assurance so that errors would not occur.

The Report of the Medical Consultants on the Diagnosis of Death to the President's Commission on Ethical Issues in Medicine and Biomedical and Behavioral Research published guidelines in 1981 (Table 1-5) that represented a distillation of practice at that time (24,25). The Commission heard philosophical, political, and religious testimony and set a day apart to hear testimony from expert witnesses in vascular surgery, neurology, and neurosurgery. It also embarked on a "small empirical study," described in their report (24,25). They attempted to develop criteria that (a) eliminated error in classifying a living individual as dead, (b) allowed as few errors as possible in classifying a dead body as alive, (c) allowed a determination to be made without unreasonable delay, and (d) were explicit, adaptable, and accessible to verification. The guidelines addressed only commonly available and verified tests,

TABLE 1-5. *President's Commission (1981)*

Unreceptive and unresponsive coma
Absent brainstem function: absent pupillary, corneal, oculocephalic, oculovestibular, oropharyn-
geal reflexes
Apnea with Pa_{CO_2} greater than 60 mmHg
Absence of posturing or seizures
Irreversibility demonstrated by establishing cause and excluding reversible conditions (sedation,
hypothermia, shock, and neuromuscular blockade)
Period of observation determined by clinical judgment
Use of cerebral blood flow tests when brainstem reflexes are not testable, sufficient cause can-
not be established, or to shorten period of observation

From "Guidelines for the determination of death: report of the medical consultants on the diagnosis of death to the President's Commission for the Study of Ethical Problems in Medicine and Biomedical and Behavioral Research." *JAMA* 1981;246:2184–2186.

were deemed advisory, and recommended consultation with other physicians. Death was defined as the "irreversible cessation of all [clinically ascertainable] functions of the entire brain including the brainstem." This was to be demonstrated by unreceptivity, unresponsivity, absent brainstem reflexes and apnea. Irreversibility was assured by (a) establishing the cause of coma, (b) excluding the possibility of recovery of any brain function (exclusion of reversible conditions), and (c) a period of observation. Apnea testing was described in detail to include preoxygenation, passive flow of oxygen during apnea, and hypercarbia of at least 60 mm Hg confirmed by arterial blood gas sampling. The report specifically indicated that true decerebrate or decorticate posturing or seizures were inconsistent with the diagnosis of death. This report was the first to include shock as a reversible condition. The period of observation was considered a matter of clinical judgment; 6 h was appropriate in uncomplicated cases with a confirmatory EEG or test of cerebral blood flow, 12 h with a well-established irreversible cause of coma without a confirmatory test, and 24 h for anoxic brain damage. Finally, the observation period could be reduced if tests showed an isoelectric EEG or absent cerebral blood flow for 10 min in an adult without drug intoxication, hypothermia, or shock.

In early 1993, the Quality Standards subcommittee of the American Academy of Neurology investigated ways to develop practice parameters using evidence-based approach to the literature. The areas of need were defined as follows: (a) unequivocal definition of clinical testing of brainstem function, (b) description of conditions that may mimic brain death, (c) clinical observations that are compatible with brain death but raised doubts in the attending physician, (d) a clear description of apnea testing procedure, and (e) critical review of the value of confirmatory laboratory tests. A comprehensive review became the basis for practice parameters (26). These guidelines, after careful review by numerous neurologists and societies, were approved by the Academy of Neurology Executive Board in 1995 (27) (Table 1-6).

The acceptance of brain death in children was advanced by publication of an ad hoc committee of Boston Children's Hospital and a special task force of neurologists and pediatricians. The recommendations included age brackets with different recommendations for time of observation and electrophysiologic tests. The time of obser-

TABLE 1-6. *American Academy of Neurology guidelines (1995)*

Demonstration of coma
Evidence for the cause of coma
Absence of confounding factors, including hypothermia, drugs, electrolyte, and endocrine disturbances
Absent brainstem reflexes
Absent motor responses
Apnea
A repeat evaluation in 6 h is advised, but the time period is considered arbitrary
Confirmatory laboratory tests are only required when specific components of the clinical testing cannot reliably be evaluated

From American Academy of Neurology Practice Parameters for Determining Brain Death in Adults (summary statement). *Neurology* 1995;45:1012–1014, with permission.

vation and use of EEG were taken from the adult Harvard Criteria (28,29). These guidelines became readily accepted although its publication was followed by an acid editorial. Freeman and Ferry (30) asserted that "'guidelines' from prestigious physicians and groups have a way of becoming dogma . . . They will be used by attorneys, hospital-governing bodies, risk management officers, medical societies, and lay groups espousing various causes." "Until better scientific data are available . . . we suggest that the diagnosis of pediatric brain death should remain a clinical one . . ." (30). Important data in newborns by Ashwal and Schneider followed after these guidelines and suggested extension to preterm and term infants (see Chapter 5) (31).

. This sequential historical review demonstrates how statutes for brain death determination have evolved over time. The currently used criteria are discussed in Chapters 4 and 5.

FURTHER REFINEMENT OF CRITERIA

Based on these definitions it is apparent that there are four elements in diagnosing death based on neurological criteria: absence of neurological function, apnea, irreversibility, and additional physiological "confirmatory" tests.

The neurological exam is used as the determinant of neurological function. To demonstrate complete loss of neurological function there should be no response to any environmental stimuli and absence of brainstem reflexes. Although the absence of respiratory drive is a brainstem reflex, the clinical, theological and emotional implications of its absence have given this function a special role in diagnosing death based on neurological criteria.

Irreversible brain damage can be demonstrated through historical or radiographic data that indicate a clear etiology or severe anatomical destruction. A variable period of observation is utilized to demonstrate irreversibility based on the natural history of the etiology. In addition, determination of irreversibility requires that no additional factors are present that could contribute to the clinical picture or mimic absence of neurological function (hypothermia, sedatives, shock).

In some situations, ancillary physiological tests are used to "confirm" absence of neurological function. Their use varies considerably, with some guidelines reserving them for situations in which the clinical evaluation cannot be completely performed, and others requiring them in all cases.

The criteria for apnea testing have changed considerably. The earliest suggested criteria did not consider whether sufficient stimulus to respiration was present before determining if apnea was present. Since patients with severe brain injuries are frequently treated with hyperventilation, initial apnea after disconnection from the ventilator may be a result of alkalosis (post-hyperventilation apnea) and not failure of central respiratory centers. Prior to the publication of the Harvard Criteria, demonstration of complete absence of respiration ranging from 5 to 30 min was suggested. Others simply stated that respiration needed to be entirely artificially maintained. The Harvard Criteria stated there must be "no movements or breathing" (6). In the NIH collaborative study, apnea was defined as the need for controlled ventilation for at least 15 min, but without strict guidelines on how to perform the apnea test (24).

Apneic diffusion oxygenation to test apnea in brain death was first reported by Milhaud from Centre Hospitalier Regional in Amiens, France in 1974 using the technique of oxygen apnea by Hirsch and Volhance described in 1905 (32). These 40 patients were tested for only 15 min to limit the development of severe hypercapnic acidosis. Marked acidosis was recognized as potentially causing cardiac arrhythmias and myocardial depression. A target $Paco_2$ was not suggested but, in a later study, a $Paco_2$ of 60 mm Hg threshold was recommended by Shafer and Caronna, surprisingly on the basis of only three patients. These patients started to breathe at levels varying from 45 to 56 mm Hg (five trials total) (33). This threshold of $Paco_2$ became accepted but was, rightly so, challenged by Ropper who found much lower breathing thresholds in four patients varying from 30 to 39 mm Hg (seven trials) (34). This $Paco_2$ threshold will be debated until a collective study in a large group of patients is published. Theoretically, too low (e.g., $Paco_2 < 30$ mm Hg) would mean insufficient stimulation to the impaired respiratory centers; too high (e.g., $Paco_2 > 100$ mm Hg) would depress possible brain function through CO_2 narcosis. The threshold of $Paco_2$ of 50 (U.K. mm Hg) or 60 (U.S. mm Hg) has been advocated in many brain death protocols without many qualms. A compromise criterion of "20 mm Hg increase above normal $Paco_2$ level" was suggested in the American Academy of Neurology guidelines (26,27). This amendment to the traditional $Paco_2$ threshold was chosen to reduce repeated testing in patients who failed to have the $Paco_2$ climb above 60 mm Hg but instead continue to border upon the "target value".

Pallis suggested not to reconnect the ventilator when family has already refused organ donation (23). This would imply discussion of brain death before completion of the tests, potentially muddling the physician-family interaction. The apnea test remains a difficult test and has never been that simple to physicians. The details about the procedure remain poorly understood, and its potential for complications when performed without adequate precautions remains substantial. The American Academy guidelines, for the first time, suggested precautionary measures and a detailed technique to facilitate the procedure. Apneic oxygen diffusion techniques remains the most reliable technique and is used in most intensive care units (26,27).

CURRENT INTERNATIONAL GUIDELINES

Neurological criteria for declaration of death have been proposed in many countries throughout the world. The acceptance of the process of declaration of death and organ donation, however, has progressed much more slowly than in the United States and may be rooted in cultural resistance to accepting neurological criteria for death. In Europe many countries have statutes that allow for the declaration of death based on neurological criteria and organ transplantation. Some, however, have only recently enacted such laws. In Germany, a law recognizing brain death as being equivalent to death was just passed in 1997 (35). South and Central American countries, including Brazil, Chile, Colombia, Venezuela, and Argentina, have medical criteria similar to the United States and legal support exists.

All three religions of the Middle East (Islam, Christianity, and Judaism; see Chapter 7) have accepted death based on neurological criteria, yet very few countries actually have legal definitions or have cadaveric donation programs. Several Asian countries (Indonesia, Malaysia, the Philippines, Singapore, and Taiwan) have laws allowing organ transplantation. Others (Bangladesh, Peoples Republic of China, South Korea, and Thailand) have no laws or laws only for kidney transplantation. Laws modeled after U.K. criteria existed in Hong Kong before it became a part of China.

Several countries have recently considered or enacted legislation that makes every citizen a potential organ donor unless they specifically indicate in writing that they do not wish to be considered a donor ("presumed consent"). Such a law exists in Brazil but is rarely enforced. Similar legislation was recently proposed in Mexico. In Belgium and France, "presumed consent" led to public unrest and now has changed into an "obligatory inquiry."

In this section, the current criteria in many countries around the world are summarized and particularly those that contrast starkly with the U.S. and U.K. position. Not much of a consensus exists with the determination procedures, but the overarching concept of brain death has been accepted.

CRITERIA IN THE UNITED STATES AND CANADA

Until recently, the responsibility for the determination of death by neurological criteria in the United States was left to individual institutions. State laws indicate that the criteria should be based on "accepted medical standards," but did not list them. The Report of the Medical Consultants on the Diagnosis of Death to the President's Commission on Ethical Issues in Medicine and Biomedical and Behavioral Research (25) considered its recommendations "advisory" and thus did not establish a national standard. Therefore each individual medical institution developed its own criteria. This led to policies that differed significantly in terms of which and how many physicians should make the determination, duration of observation, and use of physiological "confirmatory" tests.

In 1995 the Quality Standards Subcommittee of the American Academy of Neurology (AAN) published guidelines for determining brain death in adults (27). The recommendations carry the weight of guidelines rather than standards. It appears that institutional policies in the United States have been modeled using these guidelines (Table 1-6).

In 2000, the Canadian Neurocritical Care Group published Guidelines for the Diagnosis of Brain Death which closely mirror the AAN guidelines (36). The major elements included (a) established etiology and absence of potentially reversible factors, (b) coma with no response to stimulation, (c) absent brainstem reflexes, (d) apnea, (e) reassessment after a "suitable interval," and (f) absence of confounding factors. When there was inability to apply the clinical criteria they recommended demonstration of "absence of cerebral perfusion" (36) (Table 1-7).

TABLE 1-7. *The Canadian Neurocritical Care Group guidelines (2000)*

Established etiology
Absence of potentially reversible factors
Coma with no response to stimulation
Absent brainstem reflexes
Apnea
Reassessment after a suitable interval
Absence of confounding factors
Demonstration of absence of cerebral perfusion is only required when specific components of the clinical testing cannot reliably be performed

From Canadian Neurocritical Care Group. Guidelines for the diagnosis of brain death. *Can J Neurol Sci* 2000;26:64–66, with permission.

CRITERIA IN EUROPE

There is uniform acceptance of brain death across Europe. After Finland accepted brain death criteria in 1971, other countries quickly followed suit. There is fairly uniform agreement regarding the criteria for the clinical evaluation, although there is considerable variation in the use of additional physiological tests. A summary of the criteria across Europe, recently reviewed by Haupt and Rudolf (37), is found in Table 1-8. Only seven of 18 countries require a confirmatory test. Approximately half of the surveyed countries require more than one physician be involved. Additional laboratory testing is required in France, Italy, Luxembourg, and the Netherlands. Several countries have longer observation periods when "anoxia" has been the cause of brain death without much scientific justification.

CRITERIA IN ASIA, AUSTRALIA, AND NEW ZEALAND

The concept of death based on neurological criteria has not been uniformly accepted in Asia and major differences in regulations exist. In Turkey an organ harvesting law has been established and demands a cardiologist, a neurosurgeon, a neurologist, and an anesthesiologist to examine the patient, followed by confirmatory testing often requiring a combination of tests (38). Confirmatory tests are not mandatory in many third-world countries because they are not available. Unusual requirements exist (e.g., Georgia, 5-year practice in neurosciences; Iran, 12-, 24-, 36-hour observations and three physicians). In India, the Rajya Sabha passed the Transplantation of Human Organs Bill in 1993 (39). Brain death determination follows the British criteria of brainstem death but involves a panel consisting of (a) the doctor in charge of the patient, (b) the doctor in charge of the hospital where the patient was treated, (c) an independent specialist (specialty unspecified), and (d) a neurologist or neurosurgeon. The burden of proof rests with the specialist in the neurosciences with the other member confirming the diagnosis.

The little that we know about China shows in the practice of donation and brain death determination. China has no legal criteria for the determination of brain death

TABLE 1-8. *Criteria in Europe and U.K.[a]*

Country	Hours after onset	Hours to repeat testing	Number of physicians	Confirmatory test	Type of test
Austria	ND	12	1 or 2	Optional	EEG, TCD, CA
Belgium	6	ND	3	Optional	EEG ×2, EP, CA
Denmark	6 (anoxia: 24)	2; mandatory	2	Optional	CA
Finland	ND	ND	1	Optional	EEG, CA
France	ND	ND	2	Mandatory	EEG ×2, CA
Germany	ND (anoxia: 6)	12 or confirmatory test	2	Optional	EEG, EP, TCD, CA, or N
Greece	ND	8	3	Mandatory	EEG, N, CA
Italy	6 (anoxia: 24)	6	1 or more	Mandatory	EEG ×3
Luxembourg	ND	ND	1	Mandatory	EEG, EP, CA, or N
Netherlands	ND	ND	1 or more[b]	Mandatory	EEG or CA
Poland	ND	3	1	No	—
Portugal	ND	2–24; mandatory	2	Optional	EEG, EP, CA
Slovakia	ND	ND	3	Mandatory	EEG, TCD, CA
Spain	6 (anoxia: 24)	6	1	Optional	EEG or CA
Sweden	ND	2	2	Mandatory	CA (30 min apart)
Switzerland	5 (anoxia: 48)	6; mandatory	2	Helpful, but not required	EEG, EP, CA, or N
United Kingdom	6 (anoxia: 24)	Discretionary	2	No	—
Yugoslavia	ND	3	3	Optional	EEG, EP, CA

[a] All countries specifically require known etiology of coma, no intoxication, hypothermia, or shock coma, brainstem areflexia, and apnea.
[b] Neurologist or neurosurgeon.
EEG, electroencephalogram; EP, evoked potentials; CA, cerebral angiogram; N, nuclear cerebral blood flow study; TCD, transcranial Doppler; ND, not defined.
From Haupt WF, Rudolf J. European death codes: a comparison of national guidelines. *J Neurol* 1999;246: 432–437; and Garcia C, Ferro JM. European brain death codes: Portuguese guidelines [Letter]. *J Neurol* 2000;247: 140, with permission, and correspondence with neurologists from listed countries.

and there are indications of reluctance of medical staff to disconnect the ventilator. On the other hand, family members may fear being accused of murder, and some families believe that a ghost deprived of his organs may retaliate. These factors remain major obstacles. Also, although forcefully denied by Chinese officials, there are some early indications of harvesting and sale of organs from executed prisoners (39–41).

In Japan, brain death determination has been the subject of considerable controversy. In 1968, heart surgeon Wada was charged with murder after removing a heart from a patient who was allegedly not brain dead and a recipient who was allegedly not sick enough to receive a graft (Fig. 1-4). This transplant not only fostered suspicion of tampering, but the procedure by an American-trained Japanese heart surgeon (1 year after Barnard's pioneering transplant), was considered "un-Japanese." Sadly, the recipient died 83 days after the transplant. The judge dismissed the "murder case," but it was another 30 years before another heart transplant was performed. Again the case was covered with massive media attention resulting in media photographers chasing the car carrying the donor organs (42). In 1994, prior to legal support for declaration of death based on neurological criteria, kidneys were harvested from four heart-beating brain-dead donors. The situation was compounded by the involvement of the transplant surgeon in decision making regarding patient manage-

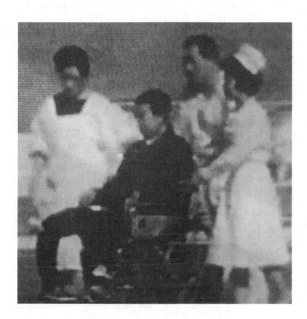

FIG. 1-4. Landmark heart transplant case that shook Japan but also was the initial stimulus for developing brain death criteria in Japan (picture showing Doctor Wada, patient, and mother at Sapporo Medical School Associated Hospital. Kindly provided by Dr. H. Takeshita).

ment and obtaining family consent. In 1985, the Ministry of Health and Welfare set up a Brain Death Advisory Council which established new brain death criteria but did not define brain death as human death (43,44). Three years later, the Japanese Medical Association voted to accept brain death as the end of human life, yet several medical specialty societies refused to accept this position. Additionally, the Ministry of Justice, the National Police Agency, and the Public Prosecutors Office all continue to resist recognition of brain death as the end of individual life (43). Due to strong resistance, the Japanese Diet has had difficulty passing a bill clearly defining neurological criteria for death. In 1997, in order to facilitate organ transplantation, Japan legalized declaration of death using neurological criteria only when the patient was to be an organ donor, creating an unfortunate double standard. Additional controversy arose in 1999 when the Japanese Health and Welfare Ministry aborted a transplantation when it was discovered that the potential donor had a ruptured tympanic membrane (45). Subsequently, the guidelines were amended to not allow brain death testing in patients with ruptured tympanic membranes (even though it in fact enhances the test) or trauma to the eyeballs.

The Japanese thinking is influenced by Confucian homilies, Buddhist traditions of care for the infirm, and Shinto, as well as other religious views, Western cultural influences, and pageantry. Confucian philosophy emphasizes that the body is a parental gift and cannot be given away. The Buddhist view emphasizes continuation of life after physical death (impermanence or *mujo*).

A cardiocentric view may be prevalent in uneducated Japanese—certainly because the word heart *(kanji)* is deeply ingrained in the written signs for center, think, and love (Fig. 1-5). More likely, the Japanese reluctant acceptance of brain death may

心   Heart

想   Think

愛   Love

中心   Center   **FIG. 1-5.** The letter *kanji* (heart) returns in think,
                                     love, and center.

have its roots in a tendency to mistrust physicians, rifts, and lingering tensions between physicians, nurses, and family in dealing with these sentimentalities and much
less from Japanese cultural thinking. Lock carefully analyzed the "Japanese brain
death problem" (43,46), and in a review, she disappointedly concluded: "What hap-
pens at the bedside of patients diagnosed as brain dead is a microcosm of an ongoing
cultural debate about what is thought to be morally appropriate in contemporary society, together with a concern about Japan's position in the global economy."

Japan has been slow to catch up with the rest of the world, but currently nearly 65%
of the Japanese accept brain death. However, 24% wish to have a donor card and 32%
want organ donation after brain death (Dr. Takeshita, personal communication).
There have been seven cases of organ transplantation since the lower Diet of the
Japanese parliament approved legalization. Currently, the Japan Organ Transplantation systems (JOT) manages the national waiting list, which includes approximately
15,000 patients waiting for kidney transplants.

The Japanese criteria have certain unique features as well. They are as follows: (a)
CT scan should detect irreparable lesions. (b) When cardiac arrest has occurred, the
cause of cardiac arrest should be known. (c) The ciliospinal reflex should be performed. (d) The apnea test should be performed after loss of seven brainstem reflexes
and after isoelectric EEG (the original Japanese criteria allowed the performance of
the apnea test before EEG). (e) Brain death determination is only allowed if intact tympanic membranes exist. (f) Children under 6 years old should be excluded, but the pe-

diatric criteria are under revision. Currently the discussion in Japan is on the type of confirmatory test in brain death and a combination may be recommended after facial or eye trauma, all in an attempt to reduce the chance of a misdiagnosis of brain death.

The Australian and New Zealand Intensive Care Society statement and guidelines on brain death were published in July 1993 and are under revision. They state that brain death determination for donation purposes should be determined by two medical practitioners. The first formal examination is performed after at least 4 h have elapsed; the second examination, 2 h after the first examination except following primary hypoxic brain injury where the first examination should not be performed until 12 h have elapsed (47,48).

CONCLUSION

In many countries, there has been acceptance of brain death. There are major differences in number of physicians, recommendations of confirmatory tests, and observation time. How these striking differences have evolved is not known, but they should be considered undesirable. Challenges to the definition of death persist in a small group of scholars. The causes for this controversy include the unique social, theological, financial, and political influences on this medical diagnosis and the lack of empirical data.

Only one study has ever been completed that attempted to prospectively derive neurological criteria for defining death—the NIH-sponsored Collaborative Study. To carry out such a study requires that brain-dead bodies be aggressively treated until there is irreversible cardiopulmonary arrest. In the current climate in the United States, Europe, and the United Kingdom, this is not ethically feasible.

Future developments should include standardization of criteria and confirmatory tests, development of more accurate confirmatory tests to assist in complex cases, and increasing the involvement of neurologic specialists in determination of brain death.

REFERENCES

1. Youngner SJ, Arnold RM, Schapiro R. *The definition of death. Contemporary Controversies.* Baltimore: Johns Hopkins University Press, 1999.
2. Bernat JL. In defense of the whole-brain concept of death. *The Hastings Center Report* 1998; 28:14–23.
3. Joynt RJ. A new look at death. *JAMA* 1984;252:680–682.
4. Pernick MS. Back from the grave: recurring controversies over defining and diagnosing death in history. In: Zaner RM, ed. *Death: beyond whole-brain criteria.* Dordrecht: Kluwer Academic Publishers, 1988:17–24.
5. Beecher HK. Definition of "life and death" for medical science and practice. *Ann NY Acad Sci* 1970; 169:471–474.
6. A definition of irreversible coma: report of the Ad Hoc Committee of the Harvard Medical School to Examine the Definition of Brain Death. *JAMA* 1968;205:337–40.
7. Lofstedt S, von Reis G. Intracranial lesions with abolished passage of x-ray contrast throughout the internal carotid arteries. *PACE* 1956;8:99–202.
8. Wertheimer P, Jouvet M, Descotes J. A propos due diagnostic de la mort du système nerveux dans les comas avec arrêt respiratoire traités par respiration artificielle. *Presse Méd* 1959;67:87–88.
9. Mollaret P, Goulon M. *Le coma dépassé (memoire preliminaire). Rev Neurol* 1959;101:3–15.

10. Schwab RS, Potts F, Mathis P. EEG as an aid in determining death in the presence of cardiac activity. *Electroencephalogr Clin Neurophysiol* 1963;15:147.
11. Murray JE. Organ transplantation: the practical possibilities. In: Wolstenholme GEW, O'Conner M, eds. *Ciba Foundation Symposium: Ethics in medical progress*. Boston: Little, Brown & Co, 1966, 54–77.
12. Appel JZ. Ethical and legal questions posed by recent advances in medicine. *JAMA* 1968; 205:513–517.
13. Beecher HK, Adams RD, Sweet WH. Procedures for the appropriate management of patients who may have supportive measures withdrawn. *JAMA* 1969;209:405.
14. Penin H, Kaufer C. The dissociated brain death. *Minn Med* 1989;51:1563–1567.
15. Adams RD, Jequier M. The brain death syndrome: hypoxemic panencephalopathy. *Schweiz Med Wochenschr* 1969;99:65–73.
16. Beecher HK. After the "Definition of irreversible coma." *N Engl J Med* 1969;281:1070–1071.
17. Becker D, Robert CMJ, Nelson JR, et al. An evaluation of the definition of cerebral death. *Neurology* 1970;20:459–462.
18. Mohandas A, Chou SN. Brain death—a clinical and pathological study. *J Neurosurg* 1971;35: 211–218.
19. Pallis C. ABC of brain death. From brain death to brain stem death. *BMJ* 1982;285:1487–1490.
20. Conference of Medical Royal Colleges and Faculties of the United Kingdom. Diagnosis of brain death. *BMJ* 1976;2:1187–1188.
21. Criteria for the diagnosis of brain stem death: review by a working group convened by the Royal College of Physicians and endorsed by the Conference of Medical Royal Colleges and Their Faculties in the United Kingdom. *J R Coll Phys Lond* 1995;29:381–382.
22. Jennett B. Brain death. *Br J Anaesth* 1981;53:1111–1119.
23. Pallis C, Harley DH. *The ABC of brainstem death*, 2nd ed. London: British Medical Journal Publishing Group, 1996.
24. An appraisal of the criteria of cerebral death, a summary statement of a collaborative study. *JAMA* 1977;237:982–986.
25. Guidelines for the determination of death: report of the medical consultants on the diagnosis of death to the President's Commission for the Study of Ethical Problems in Medicine and Biomedical and Behavioral research. *JAMA* 1981;246:2184–2186.
26. Wijdicks EFM. Determining brain death in adults. *Neurology* 1995;45:1003–1011.
27. American Academy of Neurology Practice Parameters for Determining Brain Death in Adults (summary statement). *Neurology* 1995;45:1012–1014.
28. Ad Hoc Committee on Brain Death, The Children's Hospital, Boston. Determination of brain death. *J Pediatr* 1987;110:15–19.
29. Special Task Force. Guidelines for the determination of brain death in children. *Pediatrics* 1987; 80:298–300.
30. Freeman JM, Ferry PC. New brain death guidelines in children. Further confusion. *Pediatrics* 1988; 81:301–303.
31. Ashwal S, Schneider S. Brain death in the new born. *Pediatrics* 1985;84:429–437.
32. Milhaud A, Ossart M, Gayet H, et al. L'epreuve de débrancher en oxygéne. *Test de Mort Cérèbrale, Special III* 1974;15:73–79.
33. Shafer JA, Caronna J. Duration of apnea needed to confirm brain death. *Neurology* 1978;28:661–666.
34. Ropper AH, Kennedy SK, Russel L. Apnea testing in the diagnosis of brain death. *J Neurosurg* 1981; 55:942–946.
35. Goldbeck-Wood S. Germany passes new transplant law. *BMJ* 1997;315:11.
36. Canadian Neurocritical Care Group. Guidelines for the diagnosis of brain death. *Can J Neurol Sci* 2000;26:64–66.
37. Haupt WF, Rudolf J. European brain death codes: a comparison of national guidelines. *J Neurol* 1999; 246:432–437.
38. Haberral M, Moray G, Karakayali H, et al. Ethical and legal aspects and the history of organ transplantation in Turkey. *Transplant Proc* 1996;28:382–383.
39. The Transplantation of Human Organs Bill, 1993. Bill No. LIX-C of 1992, Republic of India.
40. Chelala C. China's human organ trade highlighted by U.S. arrest of "salesman." *Lancet* 1998; 351:735.
41. Miles JA. Organ transplants in China: use of organs from executed prisoners [Letter]. *NZ Med J* 1995; 108:178.

42. BBC News Sunday; February 28, 1999. BBC online network. BBC/Health.
43. Lock M. The problem of brain death: Japanese disputes about bodies and modernity. In: Youngner SJ, Arnold RM, Schapiro R, eds. The Definition of Death: Contemporary Controversies. Baltimore: John Hopkins University Press, 1999, 239–256.
44. Takeshita H. Coma and brain death. In: Cucchiara RF, Black S, Michenfelder JD, eds. *Clinical neuroanesthesia,* 2nd ed. New York: Churchill Livingstone, 1998, 643–665.
45. Watts J. Brain-death guidelines revised in Japan. *Lancet* 1999;354:1011.
46. Lock M. Contesting the natural in Japan: moral dilemmas and technologies of dying. *Culture Med Psychiatry* 1995;19:1–38.
47. Transplantation and Anatomy Ordinance 1978. Australian Capital Territory.
48. A code of practice for transplantation of cadaveric organs. Department of Health. Wellington, New Zealand, 1987.

2

Pathophysiologic Responses to Brain Death

Eelco F. M. Wijdicks[*] and John L. D. Atkinson[†]

Departments of [*]Neurology and [†]Neurologic Surgery, Mayo Clinic, Rochester, Minnesota

Brain injury is known to affect multiple organ systems, and many brain-injured patients may have suffered systemic tissue injury before hospitalization. Brain injury due to projectiles, high-speed rapid deceleration such as motor vehicle accidents, and massive subarachnoid or intracranial hemorrhage which ultimately leads to brain death is particularly associated with systemic injuries initiated and augmented by catecholamine surge and apnea at the time of the injury. The magnitude of force and rate of change delivered to the brainstem in laboratory and clinical studies of brain injury directly correlate with two profound physiologic effects (1). One is apnea, which, by way of hypoxia, hypercarbia, and acidosis, significantly affects myocardial function. Ultimately, clinical outcome is determined by the duration and degree of apnea before mechanical ventilation is provided or spontaneous ventilation returns (2,3). The other effect is a catecholamine surge, which, under laboratory circumstances, yields catecholamine levels many fold those of resting baseline values (4,5). The degree of catecholamine surge is strongly associated with gastric mucosal ulceration, myocardial injury or necrosis, and neurogenic pulmonary edema. It may reduce the effect of cardioplegic preservation solution and precondition protocols (5).

Most pronounced in the cascade of events immediately following the defining moment of brain death is loss of tone of the vascular bed, abnormal cardiac inotropy, and cardiac arrest. Prolonged preservation of the brain-dead dehumanized body is technically possible with advanced intensive care management in some instances, but physicians are challenged with the complex ventilatory management of pulmonary edema and the treatment of frequently emerging cardiac arrhythmias, disseminated intravascular coagulation, hypotension, and hypothermia (6). These physiologic changes should be anticipated and managed in order to successfully shepherd the brain-dead person through a critical time until organ retrieval. The potential negative impact of these physiologic changes on organ utilization is substantial, as exemplified by rejection of approximately 25% of potential donor hearts and 20% of potential lung donors (7).

Understanding the pathophysiologic mechanisms after brain death may lead to effective countermeasures and, ideally, increase recovery of suitable organs. This chapter discusses the pathophysiologic impact of brain death on the function of the organs most relevant in organ procurement. A detailed account of management is given in Chapter 10 (8–11).

HYPOTHALAMIC-PITUITARY FUNCTION

Deprived of arterial perfusion, the neurosecretory neurons of the hypothalamus will die and disconnect the hypothalamic-pituitary axis. Though the pituitary gland may remain structurally intact, the pituitary stalk may be severed as a consequence of brain herniation. Herniation of the diencephalon, particularly in centrally located masses, compresses the pituitary stalk against the sharp edge of the diaphragma sellae. If the pituitary gland becomes damaged, the posterior lobe is most often involved, as reflected clinically by diabetes insipidus. Diabetes insipidus may thus be seen more often (up to 95%) in persons suffering acute mass effects; it is less common in diffuse processes such as encephalitis, meningitis, and global cerebral ischemia. The posterior lobe is usually damaged directly and not from ischemia, because it receives blood from the unaffected extradural inferior hypophyseal arteries.

A comprehensive study in 31 consecutive brain-dead persons found that 77% had clinical diabetes insipidus. Diabetes insipidus became evident with sudden polyuria and led to dehydration, hypotension, and oliguria if not treated with hormone or fluid replacement therapy (12). Because of the short half-life of antidiuretic hormone, the concentration of this hormone decreases to a barely detectable level within 15 min, and it disappears from the circulation in 4 h.

Diabetes insipidus can be diagnosed not only by polyuria but also by an increase in plasma sodium and osmolality. A decreased urinary sodium concentration (<10 mmol/L) together with hypernatremia is diagnostic, but use of mannitol and diuretics may be major confounders. Laboratory criteria for diabetes insipidus are a plasma osmolality of more than 300 mosm/L, hypotonic polyuria (more than 4 mL/kg per hour), decreased specific gravity (<1.005), and urine osmolality of less than 300 mosm/L. Diabetes insipidus will lead to dehydration, hypomagnesemia, hypokalemia, hypophosphaturia, and hypocalcemia (13). Management of diabetes insipidus is discussed in Chapter 10.

The anterior lobe of the pituitary gland is compartmentalized in the sella turcica and is usually spared in brain injury. The anterior lobe of the gland and possibly the basal part and median eminence of the hypothalamus are normally perfused through inferior and superior hypophyseal arteries from the cavernous portion of the carotid artery. The extradural source of blood supply to the pituitary may explain why normal hormone production persists in many brain-dead persons despite the arrest of intracranial flow due to increased intracranial pressure (Fig. 2-1) (14). Intact pituitary function after declaration of brain death may be due to a residual reservoir, preservation of the basal part, or the production of trophic factors from organs such as the pancreas or the placenta in brain-dead mothers. Surprisingly, the presence of normal pituitary gland function has been used as an argument against whole brain death by opponents of brain death determination (see Chapter 9).

Thyroid function should remain normal, and laboratory findings reveal a characteristic picture of "euthyroid sick syndrome." Typically, as in many critical illnesses and during fasting, serum levels of triiodothyronine (T3), total serum thyroxine (T4), free T4 index, and free T4 are decreased or borderline, but thyroid-stimulating hormone is normal. Increased concentration of reverse T3 is a consequence of transfor-

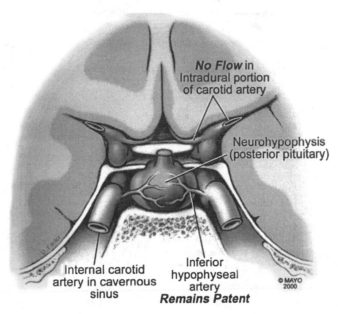

FIG. 2-1. Blood supply to the pituitary gland and its relation to the dura, emphasizing the extradural locations. (By permission of Mayo Foundation.)

mation of T4 into reverse T3. This shift occurs because, in critical illness, levels of serum proteins such as thyroid-binding globulin (TBG) decrease and binding to TBG is reduced as a result of binding-inhibiting substances (15). Novitzky and colleagues (16,17) claim that true hypothyroidism is present from decreased free T3. Indeed, free T3 may be a better marker for disturbance of the pituitary-thyroid axis. Despite evidence of a certain degree of hypothyroidism probably coinciding with a euthyroid sick syndrome, it is uncertain whether T3 infusions are systematically needed. Proponents of T3 infusion have justified its use on the basis of its effects on transsarcolemmal calcium entry, myocardial myosin, and ATPase activity, effects that may maintain ventricular contractility. In fact, studies by Novitzky and associates (16) showed a dramatic effect of T3 infusion in brain-dead hemodynamically unstable patients. A 4-h infusion of combined T3, cortisol, and insulin significantly improved circulatory status, with improvement in cardiac output and reduced need for inotropic agents. A follow-up randomized study confirmed superb hemodynamic parameters achieved with hormonal therapy (16,17). However, two other studies failed to document effects of T3 administration on myocardial contractility (18,19). Not only is the indication for T3 in question, but the appropriate dose and duration are problematic. Most studies have administered T3 only in the perioperative phase. It may also cause detrimental side effects such as cardiac arrhythmias and metabolic acidosis. Currently, T3 infusions are not typically part of a preservation protocol and could be reserved for hemodynamically unstable patients.

The noteworthy fact that circulating levels of prolactin, cortisol, growth hormone, and gonadal hormones (luteinizing hormone, follicle-stimulating hormone, testosterone) do not appreciably decrease confirms the clinical impression that panhypopituitarism is not part of brain death. One study showed that patients with severe hypotension (defined as less than 80 mm Hg systolic) did not have significantly lower serum cortisol levels (12). These persistent hormone levels are compatible with pathologic studies of the pituitary gland, which, even in patients who are on ventilators for days, may show only a few patchy infarcts with petechial hemorrhages (20). Pancreatic dysfunction may occur but is not due to pituitary insufficiency (21,22). Early insulin release is suppressed and this leads to hyperglycemia, but the effect may be indirectly related to exogenously administered epinephrine (21). Other studies suggest that pancreatic dysfunction is due to resistance to insulin from impaired receptor binding.

To summarize, although rapid depletion of vasopressin, cortisol, insulin, T4, and free T3 occurs in experimental animal models of brain death, the endocrine dysfunction in humans seems limited and is manifested mostly as isolated diabetes insipidus. Nonetheless, certain protocols exist for hormonal replacement, most notably the Papworth Hospital "hormone package," consisting of methylprednisolone, insulin, arginine vasopressin, and T3 (23). These measures can be considered if use of inotropes and volume loading does not result in a stable hemodynamic state (see Chapter 10).

MYOCARDIAL FUNCTION

A massive outpouring of plasma catecholamines may occur after a neurologic catastrophe, a hyperdynamic response that is in a sense comparable to pheochromocytoma-associated hypertensive crises (24–26). The effect of this catecholamine surge on the myocardium is still demonstrable on the electrocardiogram hours later (27,28). Pathologically, a panoply of changes may occur, including depressed and increased ST segments, inverted T waves, widened QRS complexes, and prolonged QT intervals (29,30). Multifocal myocardial contraction bands (31) and subendocardial, intraseptal, and papillary myocytolysis can be produced in baboons and rats as a result of a massive catecholamine surge, and these changes may be ameliorated by adrenalectomy. Subendocardial damage is very frequent. It may be a consequence of the shunting away of blood, which has been documented in canine heart preparations subjected to infusion of norepinephrine. In humans, similar changes occur, and these myocardial abnormalities can produce a decrease in ejection fraction, and a mosaic of wall motion abnormalities (32) (Fig. 2-2). Catecholamine-induced mechanisms of myocardial injury which have been put forward include calcium overload due to modifications of sarcolemma permeability, reperfusion injury after vasoconstriction, and cytotoxic free radicals, but currently available experiments fall short of proving their role. Most likely, coronary vasoconstriction (a Prinzmetal mechanism) causes cardiac injury and explains the pristine coronary angiograms, at least in young persons.

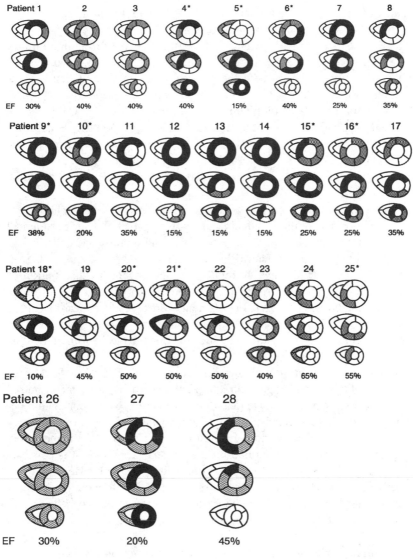

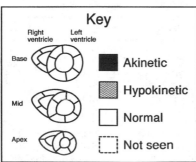

FIG. 2-2. Echocardiographic findings in 28 patients who fulfilled clinical criteria of brain death. EF, ejection fraction. (From Dujardin KS, McCully RB, Wijdicks EFM, et al. Myocardial dysfunction associated with brain death: clinical, echocardiographic, and pathologic features. *J Heart Lung Transplant* 2001 (in press), with permission of the International Society for Heart and Lung Transplantation.)

In our study of 66 consecutive brain deaths, 42% of potential heart donors were found to have echocardiographically confirmed myocardial dysfunction. Myocardial dysfunction was not predicted by cause of brain injury, time from brain injury to brain death, or need for pressor support. Similarly, electrocardiographic (ECG) abnormalities were insensitive for the detection of myocardial dysfunction, and localization studies did not match (32). In our study, only 14% of patients with myocardial dysfunction on echocardiography had prolongation of the QTc interval (>500 ms), and 14% had ST-segment depression or elevation. Ventricular arrhythmias occurred more frequently in patients with myocardial dysfunction than in those with normal function. Therefore, the onset of these arrhythmias should prompt not only treatment but also evaluation of myocardial damage with echocardiographic tests.

Spontaneous intracranial hemorrhage was associated with segmental left ventricular dysfunction, and most of these patients had sparing of the left ventricular apical region (Table 2-1). In contrast, patients with traumatic brain injury had either a segmental or a global pattern of left ventricular dysfunction (Figs. 2-2 and 2-3). Segmental myocardial dysfunction may be related to inhomogeneous distribution of adrenergic innervation of the heart, differences in sudden preload and afterload changes during catecholamine surges, or differences in myosubendocardial blood supply. A relative lack of innervation of the apex of the normal canine heart has been reported (33). Apical sparing, therefore, may indicate that the mechanism of the dysfunction is neurogenic.

Echocardiographic wall motion abnormalities may reflect reversible or irreversible myocardial injury. Although contraction band necrosis has been considered a characteristic feature of neurogenic myocardial dysfunction, a poor correlation between echocardiographically demonstrated dysfunction and pathologic findings may exist. Consequently, the myocardium may not be irreversibly damaged when echocardiographic wall motion abnormalities are present. Therefore, it is conceivable that the presence of echocardiographic abnormalities may not adversely affect cardiac function after transplantation into the recipient (7,34). In addition, a recent low-dose dobutamine stress echocardiography study in 30 brain-dead persons found, in some, reversibility of dysfunction. In this study from Japan, which allowed pro-

TABLE 2-1. *Etiology of brain injury and echocardiographic findings in 28 patients with myocardial dysfunction (from 66 consecutive patients with brain death)*

	SAH/ICH	TBI	Other
Patients, *n*	8	17	3
Age, yr	44 ± 9	25 ± 12	35 ± 6
Time from brain injury to death, h	26 ± 26	31 ± 38	136 ± 194
Ejection fraction, %	34 ± 10	36 ± 16	32 ± 14
Segmental dysfunction, *n* (%)	8 (100)	9 (53)	1 (33)
Global dysfunction, *n* (%)	0 (0)	8 (47)	2 (67)

SAH/ICH, subarachnoid or intracerebral hemorrhage; TBI, traumatic brain injury. (From Dujardin KS, McCully RB, Wijdicks EFM, et al. Myocardial dysfunction associated with brain death: clinical, echocardiographic, and pathologic features. *J Heart Lung Transplant* 2001 (in press), with permission of the International Society for Heart and Lung Transplantation.)

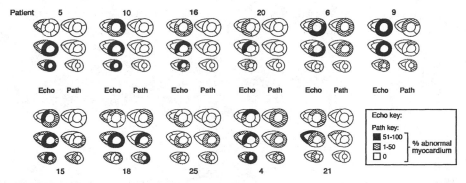

FIG. 2-3. Echocardiographic (*Echo*) and pathologic (*Path*) findings in 11 patients with myocardial dysfunction. The correlation of extent and severity of echocardiographic dysfunction with pathologic findings was poor. For ease of comparison, the pathologic groups are shown condensed: 0% abnormal myocardium (*white*), 1% to 50% (*gray*), and 51% to 100% (*black*). (From Dujardin KS, McCully RB, Wijdicks EFM, et al. Myocardial dysfunction associated with brain death: clinical, echocardiographic, and pathologic features. *J Heart Lung Transplant* 2001 (in press), with permission of the International Society for Heart and Lung Transplantation.)

longed observation of brain-dead bodies, 23% had a severe decrease in left ventricular fractional shortening, but in three of these patients contractility became normal after 7 days of observation, and levels of troponin T did not change (35).

Echocardiography is currently used routinely for screening potential donors for cardiac transplantation. Because of the often poor correlation between echocardiographic abnormalities and pathologic findings, physicians involved in the evaluation of donor candidates may need to develop more accurate techniques for identifying reversible myocardial dysfunction (7,34). A preliminary study in swine found that uptake of technetium-99m pyrophosphate could identify myocardial injury with a sensitivity of 83% and a specificity of 75% when compared with histochemical methods (36).

So too, because recent pathologic studies have been inconsistent in documenting structural myocardial abnormalities, permanent myocardial damage likely contributes little to the hemodynamic profile (37). It is more probable that hypotension is caused by the collapse of vascular tone from autonomic uncoupling, resulting in loss of baroreceptor sensitivity, invariate heart rate, and loss of blood pressure oscillations (Fig. 2-4) (38–42). Oscillations in heart rate are a product of parasympathetic and sympathetic stimuli to the heart, but the descending regulating connections from the brainstem become destroyed.

Ultimately, the heart stops in brain death. In one recent study from Taiwan, despite full cardiovascular support, 97% of 73 brain-dead bodies developed asystole in a week (43). The heart and conduction system need continuous autonomic nervous system input. When adrenergic input falls, a sudden decrease in contractility, a decrease in coronary perfusion, myocardial ischemia, and cardiac arrhythmias occur in a downward spiral. The terminal rhythms after disconnection from the ventilator are isolated atrial activity, slow junctional rhythm, sinus bradycardia, or ventricular tachycardia, but ECG activity may continue for 70 min after cardiac arrest (44,45).

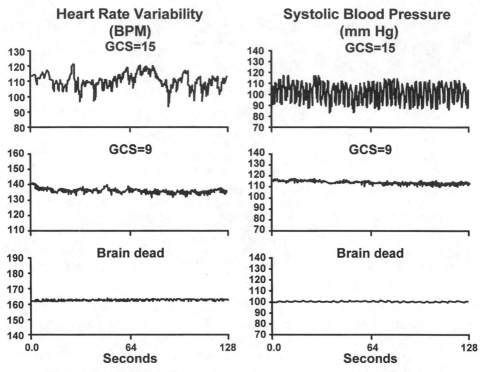

FIG. 2-4. Loss of blood pressure variability and pulse rate oscillations in brain death. **Upper row:** Normal. **Middle row:** After major insult to central nervous system. **Lower row:** Brain death. BPM, beats per minute; GCS, Glasgow Coma Scale. (Modified from Goldstein B, Toweill D, Lai S, et al. Uncoupling of the autonomic and cardiovascular systems in acute brain injury. *Am J Physiol* 1998;275:R1287–R1292, with permission of the American Physiological Society.)

PULMONARY FUNCTION

Lungs may become damaged because of trauma, aspiration pneumonitis, and fat emboli. Fiberoptic bronchoscopy may detect these abnormalities (46). Only after these conditions have been excluded should the presence of pulmonary edema be considered. Massive sympathetic stimulation may lead to extreme degrees of pulmonary vasoconstriction, and this results in pulmonary barotrauma and produces pulmonary capillary leakage of high-protein pulmonary fluid, even after vascular pressures have returned to normal (47–49). Acute left ventricular failure and a significant increase in left atrial pressure increase pulmonary artery pressure and cause a so-called blast injury (35). The mechanism of neurogenic pulmonary edema may be further elucidated by obtaining pleural fluid or analyzing pulmonary edema fluid. The protein of pulmonary edema fluid is compared with plasma protein, and ratios exceeding 0.7 suggest increased permeability. However, a recent large study found hydrostatic edema in seven of 12 patients (ratio less than 0.7) with pulmonary edema (50). Hydrostatic pulmonary edema may be seen in cases of myocardial dysfunction, but it can also be explained on the basis of profound venoconstriction due to an increase in epinephrine levels which may not be reflected in Swan-Ganz catheter measurements. This profound pulmonary venoconstriction disturbs the Starling forces in the lung, and even more fluid may be forced out when there is already increased permeability.

Considerable work has been published on the elucidation of a possible central nervous system effector site (51). Bilateral nucleus tractus solitarius (NTS) lesions produced a change in pulmonary vascular pressure and fluid influx independent of the systemic circulation. Hypothalamic lesions may contribute but through a complex regulating system that involves the NTS, the area postrema, and the ventrolateral medulla (A1 area) (49,51).

The radiologic features of pulmonary edema (Fig. 2-5) are typically a "whiteout, snowstorm pattern" but may begin in the upper lobes due to recruitment of upper lobe vessels when the pulmonary vascular bed opens. Radiologic differentiation between cardiogenic and noncardiogenic pulmonary edema or aspiration pneumonitis is very difficult in brain death. Crystalloid fluid loading may further damage the lung and increase the alveolar-arterial gradient (52). Clearance of alveolar liquid is mediated by epinephrine; therefore, beta-2-adrenergic agonist therapy (e.g., with isoproterenol or terbutaline) may theoretically accelerate reabsorption of alveolar fluid (53).

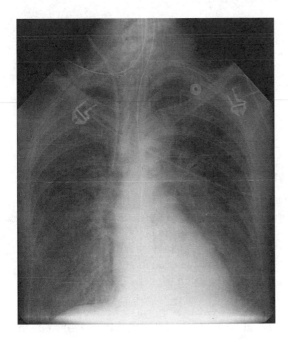

FIG. 2-5. Neurogenic pulmonary edema.

Lungs may become severely damaged from hypotension, and function may be impaired after reperfusion in a recipient. Brief hypotension, such as in the apnea test, seems an unlikely component. A mean arterial blood pressure of 40 mm Hg sustained for at least 1 h is likely needed to produce reperfusion lung injury (54). In our experience with 121 consecutive patients with brain death, true neurogenic pulmonary edema was uncommon, was easily managed with positive end-expiratory pressure, and was fully reversible. In fact, if any patients had pulmonary dysfunction, it was from aspiration or direct trauma (S. Emery and E. F. M. Wijdicks, unpublished data).

KIDNEY FUNCTION

Living-donor kidney grafts have a superb survival rate, because damage to the kidney is uncommon during procurement (55,56). One study stated that 10% of cadaver grafts may be damaged before excision but seldom irreversibly (57). Often brief periods of hypotension are implicated.

Dopamine may reduce allograft rejection (58), not only through support of blood pressure but possibly also through more complex mechanisms that inhibit expression of adhesion molecules, which are required for leukocyte migration into the graft, to produce acute rejection (59).

LIVER FUNCTION

Very few experimental studies have evaluated liver function in brain-dead donors, but changes appear as early as 3 h after the clinical determination of brain death. Vacuolization in the vicinity of sinusoids and early disintegration of mitochondria and endoplasmic reticulin are noted on electron microscopy, along with reduced bile production and stagnated leukocytes in sinusoids; endothelial cells, however, remain intact. An increase in interleukin-6 levels may induce expression of adhesion molecules as in the kidney (60).

COAGULOPATHY

Disseminated intravascular coagulation may occur when brain-dead bodies are maintained for more than 2 days. Multiple causes of this disorder may be put forward, and indeed it is more common in multitraumatized patients, who are at risk for fat emboli, and in female patients with complicated pregnancy causing embolization of amniotic fluid. Head injury and gunshot wounds to the head may cause entry of brain tissue or its thromboplastin into capillaries and elicit a triggering mechanism for intravascular coagulation. Generally, however, the overwhelming amount of thromboplastin derived from total brain necrosis readily causes fibrin deposition in the microcirculation, resulting in laboratory abnormalities such as reduced fibrinogen levels, prolonged partial thromboplastin time, and thrombocytopenia. Replacement of blood factors by means of fresh frozen plasma may not prevent microthrombi deposits in donor organs. The clinical relevance of microthrombi for graft function is unclear, but most studies appear to show no effect on liver, pancreas, and kidney graft function (61,62).

MAINTENANCE OF THE BRAIN-DEAD BODY

Although it is extremely difficult to maintain hemodynamic stability after brain death, the inevitable cardiac arrest is postponed in some instances. At least 50 cases have been unearthed from the medical literature and news media in which there was prolonged survival and the diagnosis seemed clear (63). In these extraordinary examples—related to alleged religious or cultural objections (see Chapter 7), or to physicians' capitulation to the unreasonable demands of family members who refused to recognize death in a child or young adult—the dead bodies were supported by mechanical ventilation and continuous infusion of vasopressin and pressor agents, including dopamine and norepinephrine.

Our own experience with cases in which prolonged support was reluctantly given is typically a rapid downward spiralling of vital functions. However, as long as the circulation, oxygenation, and endocrine function remain intact, these immobile, physiologically unchallenged bodies can possibly be preserved. Preservation for a mean of 23 days was reported by Yoshioka et al. (64) with the use of infusions of vasopressin (1–2 units/h) and adrenaline (0.5 mg/kg). Many organs have their own "pacemakers" and, when nutrition and oxygen are provided, will go on functioning. The vital functions, however, do not become entirely automatic. More typical is a gradual deterioration over days and the need for progressively increasing doses of inotropic agents and vasopressin until cardiac arrest occurs (Fig. 2-6).

Most impressive is the maintenance of a pregnant brain-dead woman for up to 15 weeks, from 17 to 32 weeks of gestation, but such anecdotal cases do not alter the fact that the efforts to use the mother's body as an "incubator" for maturation of the fetus fail in the vast majority of cases. The financial cost of maintaining a pregnant dead mother for weeks is enormous, an estimated $1,000 per day, amounting to $2 million per successful outcome (61). Further discussion of the ethical problems posed by this difficult situation are provided by Bernat in Chapter 9.

CONCLUSION

Massive activation of the sympathetic nervous system may be detrimental to the heart and lungs; other organs remain unharmed. Hemodynamic status may also deteriorate from loss of vascular tone and also as a result of hypotension and hypovolemia, which are initially reversible but progress unrelentingly. Brain death leads to progressive deterioration of possible donor organs. The initial major management

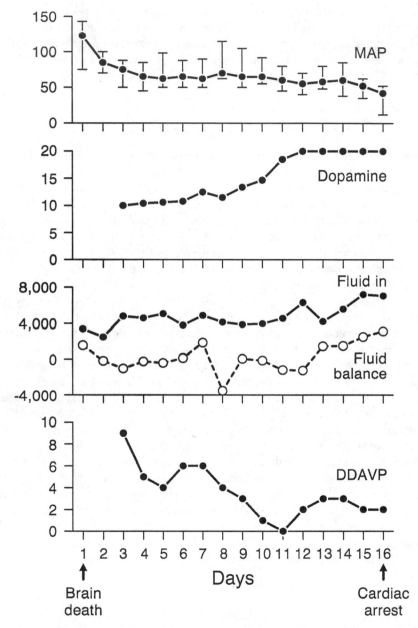

FIG. 2-6. Brain-dead patient with prolonged support. Note gradual decline of MAP and increase in dopamine dosage and fluid intake. MAP, mean arterial pressure (mm Hg); dopamine dosage, μg/kg per minute; fluid intake at balance, liters; DDAVP, vasopressin, total daily dose in μg. (From Wijdicks EFM, Bernat JL. Response to chronic "brain death": meta-analysis and conceptual consequences [Letter]. *Neurology* 1999;53:1369–1370, with permission of the American Academy of Neurology.)

concerns deal with hypotension (from collapse of arterial tone), invariate heart rate (loss of autonomic control), and polyuria (diabetes insipidus). A barrage of systemic problems may come later. The challenge is to keep vital organs in perfect condition for transplantation after the brain has died.

REFERENCES

1. Atkinson JL. The neglected prehospital phase of head injury: apnea and catecholamine surge. *Mayo Clin Proc* 2000;75:37–47.
2. Denny-Brown D, Russell WR. Experimental cerebral concussion. *Brain* 1941;64:93–164.
3. Walker AE, Kollros JJ, Case TJ. Physiological basis of concussion. *J Neurosurg* 1944;1:103–116.
4. Rosner MJ, Newsome HH, Becker DP. Mechanical brain injury: the sympathoadrenal response. *J Neurosurg* 1984;61:76–86.
5. Kirsch M, Farhat F, Garnier JP, et al. Acute brain death abolishes the cardioprotective effects of ischemic preconditioning in the rabbit. *Transplantation* 2000;69:2013–2019.
6. Scheinkestel CD, Tuxen DV, Cooper DJ, et al. Medical management of the (potential) organ donor. *Anaesth Intensive Care* 1995;23:51–59.
7. Boucek MM, Mathis CM, Kanakriyeh MS, et al. Donor shortage: use of the dysfunctional donor heart. *J Heart Lung Transplant* 1993;12:S186–S190.
8. Atkinson JL, Anderson RE, Murray MJ. The early critical phase of severe head injury: importance of apnea and dysfunctional respiration. *J Trauma* 1998;45:941–945.
9. Sullivan HG, Martinez J, Becker DP, et al. Fluid-percussion model of mechanical brain injury in the cat. *J Neurosurg* 1976;45:520–534.
10. Gennarelli TA. Head injury in man and experimental animals: clinical aspects. *Acta Neurochir Suppl* 1983;32:1–13.
11. Carey ME, Sarna GS, Farrell JB, et al. Experimental missile wound to the brain. *J Neurosurg* 1989;71:754–764.
12. Howlett TA, Keogh AM, Perry L, et al. Anterior and posterior pituitary function in brain-stem-dead donors. A possible role for hormonal replacement therapy. *Transplantation* 1989;47:828–834.
13. Power BM, Van Heerden PV. The physiological changes associated with brain death–current concepts and implications for treatment of the brain dead organ donor. *Anaesth Intensive Care* 1995;23:26–36.
14. Gramm HJ, Meinhold H, Bickel U, et al. Acute endocrine failure after brain death? *Transplantation* 1992;54:851–857.
15. Cooper DK, Basker M. Physiologic changes following brain death. *Transplant Proc* 1999;31:1001–1002.
16. Novitzky D, Cooper DK, Morrell D, et al. Change from aerobic to anaerobic metabolism after brain death, and reversal following triiodothyronine therapy. *Transplantation* 1988;45:32–36.
17. Novitzky D, Cooper DK, Reichart B. Hemodynamic and metabolic responses to hormonal therapy in brain-dead potential organ donors. *Transplantation* 1987;43:852–854.
18. Randell TT, Hockerstedt KA. Triiodothyronine treatment in brain-dead multiorgan donors—a controlled study. *Transplantation* 1992;54:736–738.
19. Goarin JP, Cohen S, Riou B, et al. The effects of triiodothyronine on hemodynamic status and cardiac function in potential heart donors. *Anesth Analg* 1996;83:41–47.
20. McCormick WF, Halmi NS. The hypophysis in patients with coma depasse ("respirator brain"). *Am J Clin Pathol* 1970;54:374–383.
21. Masson F, Thicoipe M, Gin H, et al. The endocrine pancreas in brain-dead donors. A prospective study in 25 patients. *Transplantation* 1993;56:363–367.
22. Yoshida H, Hiraide A, Yoshioka T, et al. Transient suppression of pancreatic endocrine function in patients following brain death. *Clin Transpl* 1996;10:28–33.
23. Wheeldon DR, Potter CD, Oduro A, et al. Transforming the "unacceptable" donor: outcomes from the adoption of a standardized donor management technique. *J Heart Lung Transplant* 1995;14:734–742.
24. Connor RC. Heart damage associated with intracranial lesions. *BMJ* 1968;3:29–31.
25. Doshi R, Neil-Dwyer G. A clinicopathological study of patients following a subarachnoid hemorrhage. *J Neurosurg* 1980;52:295–301.
26. Jiang JP, Downing SE. Catecholamine cardiomyopathy: review and analysis of pathogenetic mechanisms. *Yale J Biol Med* 1990;63:581–591.

27. Pollick C, Cujec B, Parker S, et al. Left ventricular wall motion abnormalities in subarachnoid hemorrhage: an echocardiographic study. *J Am Coll Cardiol* 1988;12:600–605.
28. Seiler C, Laske A, Gallino A, et al. Echocardiographic evaluation of left ventricular wall motion before and after heart transplantation. *J Heart Lung Transplant* 1992;11:867–874.
29. Mayer SA, LiMandri G, Sherman D, et al. Electrocardiographic markers of abnormal left ventricular wall motion in acute subarachnoid hemorrhage. *J Neurosurg* 1995;83:889–896.
30. Kono T, Morita H, Kuroiwa T, et al. Left ventricular wall abnormalities in patients with subarachnoid hemorrhage: neurogenic stunned myocardium. *J Am Coll Cardiol* 1994;24:636–640.
31. Karch SB, Billingham ME. Myocardial contraction bands revisited. *Hum Pathol* 1986;17:9–13.
32. Dujardin KS, McCully RB, Wijdicks EFM, et al. Myocardial dysfunction associated with brain death: clinical, echocardiographic, and pathologic features. *J Heart Lung Transplant* 2001 (in press).
33. Dae MW, O'Connell JW, Botvinick EH, et al. Scintigraphic assessment of regional cardiac adrenergic innervation. *Circulation* 1989;79:634–644.
34. Doroshow RW, Ashwal S, Saukel GW. Availability and selection of donors for pediatric heart transplantation. *J Heart Lung Transplant* 1995;14:52–58.
35. Taniguchi S, Kitamura S, Kawachi K, et al. Effects of hormonal supplements on the maintenance of cardiac function in potential donor patients after cerebral death. *Eur J Cardiothorac Surg* 1992;6:96–101.
36. Satur CM, Doyle D, Darracott-Cankovic S, et al. Can technetium-99m pyrophosphate be used to quantify myocardial injury in donor hearts? *Ann Thorac Surg* 1999;68:2225–2230.
37. Bruinsma GJ, Nederhoff MG, Geertman HJ, et al. Acute increase of myocardial workload, hemodynamic instability, and myocardial histological changes induced by brain death in the cat. *J Surg Res* 1997;68:7–15.
38. Herijgers P, Borgers M, Flameng W. The effect of brain death on cardiovascular function in rats. Part I. Is the heart damaged? *Cardiovasc Res* 1998;38:98–106.
39. Herijgers P, Flameng W. The effect of brain death on cardiovascular function in rats. Part II. The cause of the *in vivo* haemodynamic changes. *Cardiovasc Res* 1998;38:107–115.
40. Goldstein B, Toweill D, Lai S, et al. Uncoupling of the autonomic and cardiovascular systems in acute brain injury. *Am J Physiol* 1998;275:R1287–R1292.
41. Freitas J, Puig J, Rocha AP, et al. Heart rate variability in brain death. *Clin Auton Res* 1996;6:141–146.
42. Rapenne T, Moreau D, Lenfant F, et al. Could heart rate variability analysis become an early predictor of imminent brain death? A pilot study. *Anesth Analg* 2000;91:329–336.
43. Hung TP, Chen ST. Prognosis of deeply comatose patients on ventilators. *J Neurol Neurosurg Psychiatry* 1995;58:75–80.
44. Ouaknine G. Bedside procedures in the diagnosis of brain death. *Resuscitation* 1975;4:159–177.
45. Logigian EL, Ropper AH. Terminal electrocardiographic changes in brain-dead patients. *Neurology* 1985;35:915–918.
46. Riou B, Guesde R, Jacquens Y, et al. Fiberoptic bronchoscopy in brain-dead organ donors. *Am J Respir Crit Care Med* 1994;150:558–560.
47. Maron MB, Holcomb PH, Dawson CA, et al. Edema development and recovery in neurogenic pulmonary edema. *J Appl Physiol* 1994;77:1155–1163.
48. Novitzky D, Wicomb WN, Rose AG, et al. Pathophysiology of pulmonary edema following experimental brain death in the chacma baboon. *Ann Thorac Surg* 1987;43:288–294.
49. Simon RP. Neurogenic pulmonary edema. *Neurol Clin* 1993;11:309–323.
50. Smith WS, Matthay MA. Evidence for a hydrostatic mechanism in human neurogenic pulmonary edema. *Chest* 1997;111:1326–1333.
51. Simon RP, Gean-Marton AD, Sander JE. Medullary lesion inducing pulmonary edema: a magnetic resonance imaging study. *Ann Neurol* 1991;30:727–730.
52. Pennefather SH, Bullock RE, Dark JH. The effect of fluid therapy on alveolar arterial oxygen gradient in brain-dead organ donors. *Transplantation* 1993;56:1418–1422.
53. Lane SM, Maender KC, Awender NE, et al. Adrenal epinephrine increases alveolar liquid clearance in a canine model of neurogenic pulmonary edema. *Am J Respir Crit Care Med* 1998;158:760–768.
54. Tremblay LN, Yamashiro T, DeCampos KN, et al. Effect of hypotension preceding death on the function of lungs from donors with nonbeating hearts. *J Heart Lung Transplant* 1996;15:260–268.
55. Agodoa LY, Eggers PW. Renal replacement therapy in the United States: data from the United States Renal Data System. *Am J Kidney Dis* 1995;25:119–133.
56. Terasaki PI, Cecka JM, Gjertson DW, et al. High survival rates of kidney transplants from spousal and living unrelated donors. *N Engl J Med* 1995;333:333–336.

57. Halloran PF, Aprile MA, Farewell V, et al. Early function as the principal correlate of graft survival. A multivariate analysis of 200 cadaveric renal transplants treated with a protocol incorporating anti-lymphocyte globulin and cyclosporine. *Transplantation* 1988;46:223–228.
58. Schnuelle P, Lorenz D, Mueller A, et al. Donor catecholamine use reduces acute allograft rejection and improves graft survival after cadaveric renal transplantation. *Kidney Int* 1999;56:738–746.
59. Carlos TM, Clark RS, Franicola-Higgins D, et al. Expression of endothelial adhesion molecules and recruitment of neutrophils after traumatic brain injury in rats. *J Leukoc Biol* 1997;61:279–285.
60. Okamoto S, Corso CO, Kondo T, et al. Changes in hepatic microcirculation and histomorphology in brain-dead organ donors: an experimental study in rats. *Eur J Surg* 1999;165:759–766.
61. Cheng SS, Pinson CW, Lopez RR, et al. Effect of donor-disseminated intravascular coagulation in liver transplantation. *Arch Surg* 1991;126:1292–1296.
62. Hefty TR, Cotterell LW, Fraser SC, et al. Disseminated intravascular coagulation in cadaveric organ donors. Incidence and effect on renal transplantation. *Transplantation* 1993;55:442–443.
63. Shewmon DA. Chronic "brain death": meta-analysis and conceptual consequences. *Neurology* 1998; 51:1538–1545.
64. Yoshioka T, Sugimoto H, Uenishi M, et al. Prolonged hemodynamic maintenance by the combined administration of vasopressin and epinephrine in brain death: a clinical study. *Neurosurgery* 1986; 18:565–567.

3

Neuropathology of Brain Death

Jan E. Leestma

Chicago Institute of Neurosurgery and Neuroresearch, Chicago, Illinois

A new pathologic phenomenon unravelled after the development of an effective ar-tificial respiration and other advances in medical technology. When, after many days, ventilation in these comatose, nonbreathing individuals was terminated and an au-topsy performed, a hitherto unobserved specimen, conveniently termed "respirator brain," was encountered. In some notable cases, when the cranium was opened, a liq-uefied brain poured forth. To many pathologists of the time, it was thought that some infectious process, possibly viral, might be responsible.

Preceding and paralleling the observations noted above was the question of when it was appropriate to terminate artificial ventilation in these patients, essenti-ally causing cardiac arrest (1–4). The main practical considerations at the time were as follows: what measures of brain function or lack thereof were reliably predic-tive of irreversible brain dysfunction and could justify termination of life support measures?

As alluded to in Chapter 1, these considerations prompted the National Institutes of Health to organize and sponsor a national study to resolve the issues of appropri-ate criteria for termination of life support, declaring "brain death." This study, the NIH Collaborative Study on Cerebral Survival, headed by A. E. Walker, resolved to study about 600 cases in nine major medical centers across the United States from clinical, neurophysiological, and pathological perspectives (5).

In the course of the Collaborative Study, a number of technologies were evalu-ated as potentially having utility in predicting an unfavorable outcome or survival. These included analysis of electroencephalographic patterns and evaluation of several methods of measuring cerebral blood flow and neuropathological studies, all of which generated a rich literature and much valuable information (6,7). The legacy of this study was that state legislatures across the United States have now all adopted, at the very least, statutes that recognize the validity of brain death as a criterion for termination of life support. In this chapter, I discuss the processes that may affect the type of pathologic changes, and gross and microscopic patho-logic appearances, and, when applicable, make reference to forensic considerations as well.

There are several physiological systems that interact with one another to maintain a complex dynamic intracranial equilibrium quite apart from neural function. These are the mechanisms involved in regulation of pressure–volume equilibria; regulation of vascular perfusion (pressure and blood flow); and regulation of the so-called blood–brain barrier and intercellular compartments. A brief review of these systems that are involved in brain death is discussed below. This section is a slight detour from the chapter's main theme but important for a critical understanding.

PATHOPHYSIOLOGY OF CATASTROPHIC BRAIN LESIONS

The physiology of intracranial pressure and intracranial volume regulation have been the subject of a great deal of research that has gone a long way toward defining the parameters of this important system and to elucidate the consequences of failures in this system. These changes are central to the problem inherent in the development of brain death and the respirator brain (8).

From a basic point of view, total intracranial volume (V_T) is a function of the following elements:

$$V_T = V_{Bl} + V_{CSF} + V_{Br} + V_{H_2O} + V_X$$

Where V_T is the total intracranial volume, V_{Bl} is the intracranial volume contribution of blood in the brain at any point in time, V_{CSF} is the intracranial volume contribution of cerebrospinal fluid (CSF) in the ventricles and in the subarachnoid space over the brain, V_{Br} is the volume contribution of the brain tissue mass, V_{H_2O} is the volume contribution of intracellular and intercellular water in the brain, and V_X is the volume contribution of a possible tumor, hematoma, or other mass lesion not normally present.

In a normal, steady state, all components that make up V_T are in equilibrium and vary only slightly giving rise to a relatively constant intracranial pressure of about 8 to 10 mm Hg. This pressure range constantly varies within normal parameters in a pulsatile fashion, although the course of this pulsation is still open to question (9,10).

Cerebrospinal Fluid Physiology

CSF is generally thought of as being produced in the choroid plexuses of the brain's ventricles, but this source may actually account for only half of the CSF, the rest coming from other sources including the brain itself. In any case, CSF production has been measured at about 0.3 to 0.4 mL/min (or about 500 mL/day) in an adult. Another expression of CSF dynamics is that the total instantaneous volume of CSF is totally replaced every 8 h, or three to four times per day (11).

Like the origin of CSF, its absorption is not completely understood. CSF production is relatively independent of intracranial pressure except when intracranial pressure is significantly elevated over time (12). CSF production may also be diminished if there is sufficient decrease in blood flow through the choroid plexuses (12). Absorption of CSF is pressure mediated, increasing as intracranial pressure rises and decreasing when intracranial pressure falls. Classically the arachnoidal granulations along the superior sagittal sinus are thought to account for most of the absorption, but so-called "bulk" flow through the ependyma into the interstitial space may be as important. There may even be significant absorption via the choroid plexuses (13). Furthermore, the dural sheaths around spinal and cranial nerves are probably also involved in CSF absorption, a phenomenon that is probably vitally important once mass lesions have depleted intracranial CSF volume, leaving only the spinal sac CSF to support the upper mass of brain above the foramen magnum. There are many factors that can interfere with CSF absorption. These include the presence of blood or elevated protein or inflammatory exudates in the subarachnoid space (11).

CSF that is produced by the choroid plexuses, and other sources within the brain, must have a means of egress out of the interior of the brain. Critical outflow channels, that may become compromised by masses or shifts of the brain are: the foramina of Munro; the cerebral aqueduct (of Sylvius); the lateral foramina of Luschka and midline foramen of Magendie in the 4th ventricle. Once CSF has exited the interior of the brain it must be able to flow over the surface of the brain in the subarachnoid space, and up and down in the spinal sac. The most important factors in this delicate equilibrium between CSF production and absorption are: the rate of CSF production; the ability of the cisterns, subarachnoid space, and ventricular chambers to "store" or release CSF (capacitance function); the impedance to flow occasioned by the size of the various foramina, and the impedance of the subarachnoid space as well as the impedance of the various absorptive structures. This latter function seems most dependent on the level of venous pressure in the superior sagittal sinus (8,14). All of these parameters interact to determine intracranial pressure and a perturbation of any one of them can upset the equilibrium.

Another important aspect of the pressure–volume dynamic is brain compliance (8). In practical terms, compliance is the rate of change of brain (or intracranial) volume with respect to changes in intracranial pressure or vice versa. Experimental observations have defined many parameters of this relationship that appears to display, in a simplified fashion, two phases. When intracranial pressure or volume is abnormally low and then gradually increases, volume or pressure differentially increases rapidly at first but then asymptotically decrements to a plateau of the normal steady state. In this domain, incremental pressure or volume changes result in almost no change in differential intracranial volume or pressure. Beyond this plateau, however, even incremental changes in either volume or pressure cause an exponential rise in the other parameter. From the perspective of time, it should be obvious that there is a relatively constant domain of function that has a time course, during which changes may not be appreciated clinically but once certain parameters are exceeded, clinical symptoms may evolve precipitously as intracranial pressure rises.

Cerebrovascular Regulation

Just as pressure and volume have a complex relationship, so do global and regional cerebral flow, oxygen and carbon dioxide levels, as well as glucose levels in blood. It appears that a major portion of control of cerebral blood flow is mediated locally by a presumably "autoregulatory" mechanism of vasodilatation and constriction and shunting in response to local or global blood pressure and metabolic demands for blood flow. This function is preserved when variations in peripheral blood pressure do not result in concomitant variations in cerebral blood flow. It is well known that increases of $Paco_2$ lead to vasodilatation, and decrease may result in vasoconstriction, but not always in a predictable or uniform manner. When autoregulation fails because of global ischemia or the complex effects of traumatic brain injury, cerebral perfusion varies widely along with systemic blood pressure and may result in increased intracranial pressure and vasogenic edema. Cerebrovascular autoregulation appears to be more vulnerable to disruption in response to trauma in children younger than about 5 years of age (14–18), though some have suggested that traumatic edema in infants and children occurs independent of a disorder of vascular autoregulation (17,18). In adults the expected overall response to head trauma is a decrease in cerebral blood flow, whereas in children trauma may result in increased cerebral blood flow. In certain circumstances this may result in a condition described as "malignant" cerebral edema (15), which carries a high mortality rate despite treatment.

The normal rate of cerebral blood flow is about 57 mL/min per 100 g of brain (19,20), 800 mL/min for the whole brain. At all times, the brain requires about 3.5 mL/min/100 g of oxygen (about 50 mL/min whole brain) and, on average, 5.5 mg/min/100 g of glucose (77 mg/min whole brain). However, there are regional differences in blood flow and oxygen consumption, and they can be documented using positron emission tomography, single photon emission computed tomography, or functional magnetic resonance imaging (19). For example, gray matter has four to five times the blood flow, and metabolic rate, of white matter.

Selective Vulnerability

Metabolic vulnerability of neurons due to deprivation of oxygen, glucose or blood supply is not uniform (21). Among those most vulnerable are the neurons of the Sommer's sector of the hippocampus, cerebellar Purkinje cells, neurons of the dentate nuclei of the cerebellum, larger neocortical neurons, larger neurons of the basal ganglia, and others. More resistant to insults are the neurons of the spinal cord, smaller neurons of the cortex, much of the thalamus, neurons of the fascia dentata of the hippocampus, and others. One of the mechanisms involved in attempting balancing functional activity and the metabolic blood flow needs in the brain is through cerebrovascular autoregulation (17–19). The importance of this process to the issue of selective vulnerability is that in certain pathological circumstances that include the presence of mass lesions, global ischemia, or multifocal processes such as diffuse axonal injury (DAI) microcirculatory differences in perfusion from one region of the brain to another may exist. This may be due to the relevant pathological process that can account for regional differences in neuronal and axonal preservation or damage (22).

In a catastrophic failure of circulation that is inherent to the evolution of brain death, it is inevitable that not all areas of the brain are affected equally and uniformly as the process evolves. This nonuniformity is manifested physiologically and pathologically. From a clinical point of view, one can regularly observe in the brain-dying patient preservation of certain reflexes in the face of absence of other key indicators of brain function (7). In addition, electroencephalographic studies may show waxing and waning levels of electrophysiological brain function and even preservation of some function in the face of apparent widespread destruction of the brain at autopsy (6,23,24).

A further process that may affect the degree of pathological changes in a dead brain is the influence in the evolution of the effects of hypoxia-ischemia in the acutely injured as opposed to the chronically injured brain. Lindenberg (25,26) noted that the brains of acutely injured individuals who died at varying intervals after a catastrophic event such as traumatic brain injury, stroke, or gunshot wounds tended to show more severe changes in the brain and were associated with hypoxia-ischemia and postmortem artifacts than brains of individuals who died after a more chronic course. While this process has yet to be explained, it should be considered in the interpretation of pathological findings in some cases of brain death when aging and dating issues are important.

Blood–Brain Barrier and Edema

The brain has a very small extracellular space and a special system that regulates intracellular water. The main components of this system, referred to as the blood–brain barrier, are brain capillaries that have a structure different from most capillaries elsewhere in the body. Endothelial junctions are very tight and limit the passage of molecules through them into the extracellular space (27,28). Additionally, virtually all brain capillaries are completely covered by astrocytic foot processes that further serve to regulate and limit passage of blood-borne components into the brain's substance. Disruptions of virtually any component of the barrier system will result in passage of water, and possibly other substances into the brain, causing cerebral edema. To be sure there are compensatory mechanisms that can transport and absorb water, but these systems can be disrupted or overwhelmed by physical forces, and metabolic parameters.

Perturbations of blood flow, oxygen or glucose supply result in rapid and profound loss of neural as well as blood–brain barrier function. For example, total interruption of blood supply to the brain results in loss of consciousness in about one circulation time, i.e., 10 s. This means that the brain can totally exhaust its supply lines very rapidly. Even if cerebral blood flow is reduced to half its normal level, unconsciousness will result, though not as rapidly as in total cessation (20). At the same time that consciousness is disrupted, but in a much less predictable or constant manner, the blood–brain barrier is affected, resulting in influx of water into the extracellular environment of the brain (vasogenic edema), and neurons and probably glial cells may undergo metabolically mediated intracellular edema (cytotoxic edema). In combination, brain edema increases brain volume and potentially intracranial pressure (11,29,30).

From the foregoing it is clear that there are many interlocking homeostatic mechanisms in the brain. When there has been a major local or a global insult the effects of such an insult will impact all of these mechanisms in varying degrees. However, when there is a major episode of traumatic brain injury, hemorrhage in the brain, evolving mass, acute severe metabolic derangement, circulatory or respiratory fail-

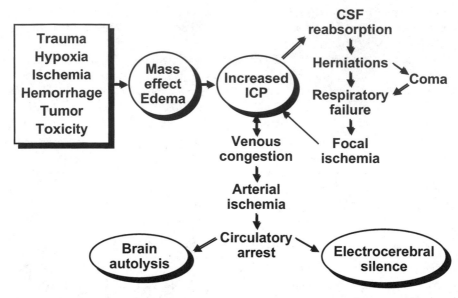

FIG. 3-1. The mechanism of brain death. The inciting process (trauma, hypoxia, ischemia, etc.) generates cerebral edema or mass effect. This, in turn, may alter intracranial pressure/volume equilibrium, leading to increased intracranial pressure. The main compensatory mechanism to restore equilibrium is cerebrospinal fluid (CSF) reabsorption. When most of the CSF has been reabsorbed and the brain has shifted to occupy former collections of CSF, herniation will have occurred and intracranial pressure may rise again, possibly driving blood from the brain, locally or globally. Brain herniation leads to loss of consciousness, coma, and eventually respiratory failure that produces more brain ischemia and further rise in intracranial pressure. Venous outflow may be compromised, causing an even greater rise in intracranial pressure that may exceed arterial perfusion pressure. At this point, cerebral circulation may be severely disturbed or cease entirely leading to electrocerebral silence. Once circulation ceases, within minutes the brain becomes irreversibly damaged and begins to undergo cellular necrosis, leading to autolysis.

ure, the effect on the brain in terms of the time course of phenomena and precise outcomes cannot be accurately predicted. In general, when the compensatory mechanisms fail irreversibly the outcome is brain death. For purposes of establishing an overview, recognizing there are many exceptions and complexities not illustrated, the general mechanism of brain death is illustrated in Figure 3-1.

NEUROPATHOLOGY IN BRAIN DEATH

If one were to examine the brain of an individual who rapidly dies from cardiac arrest within hours of occurrence, the pathological appearance might not be striking, showing little more than cerebral edema. In intracranial causes of death, one will find the immediate and secondary effects of the lesion. For example, in an acute subdural hematoma there would be effacement of the brain immediately beneath the hematoma with possible vasocongestion or perivascular hemorrhage. Edema may be present due to endothelial ischemia and reperfusion as intracranial and local pres-

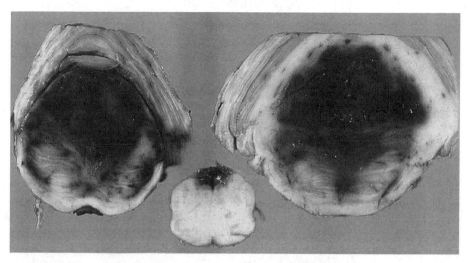

FIG. 3-2. Cross sections of the brainstem from a patient who developed an acute basal ganglion hypertensive hemorrhage and died within about 6 h of the hemorrhage but did not fulfill clinical criteria of brain death, illustrate the typical pattern of a large Duret hemorrhage. Note the central hemorrhage in the midbrain (left), the tegmentum of the pons (right), but no hemorrhage into the medulla (center), except into the 4th ventricle. Often elongation and compression are seen as well. Compare with Figure 6-2, which shows a primary traumatic lesion as well as medulla oblongata sparing. Both figures illustrate dramatic damage to the brainstem but with isolated medulla oblongata preservation, which may be observed clinically.

sures waxed and waned and there are volume-shift effects on the brain. If the hematoma were large enough and evolved quickly, there may be secondary brainstem herniation hemorrhages (Duret hemorrhages) in the pons and midbrain (Fig. 3-2). Microscopically there might also be very little other than edema present in other immediately noninvolved areas of the brain. The neuropathologic changes in patients fulfilling clinical criteria of brain death may be much more dramatic.

Pathological Characteristics of Respirator Brain

In the course of time, once intracranial blood flow has arrested, the brain will increasingly take on a dusky, congested, discolored appearance and become progressively more and more soft, eventually liquefying (Fig. 3-3). These changes may not be uniform. One of the earliest affected portions of the brain is the upper brainstem: diencephalon and cerebellum. These areas may be nearly liquefied although the cerebrum may appear relatively intact. There may be patchy involvement of the brainstem with relative preservation of the medulla. As a rule, the spinal cord is preserved but at times softness and duskiness of the cervical cord and medulla can occur. In these cases anastomoses that provide collateral circulation from below (anterior and other spinal arteries via radicular arteries) may be deficient resulting in a watershed area for the upper cord and medulla which are mostly perfused from the intracranial circulation.

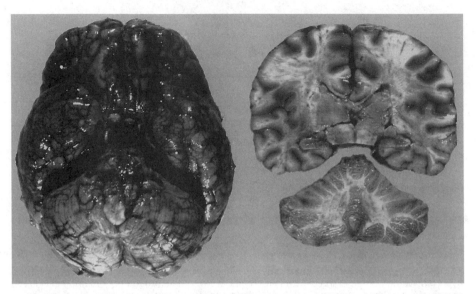

FIG. 3-3. A typical advanced respirator brain (3 days on respirator) is illustrated in a basal view and a coronal section with corresponding section of the cerebellum. Note the highly congested, dark appearance of the brain (left). On the right, the duskiness is mostly superficial, confined to the cortex where extensive extravasation of blood into the cortex was noted microscopically. The white matter was soft and also somewhat discolored, as was the cerebellum. Cause of death was anoxic ischemic encephalopathy after cardiac resuscitation.

The evolution to the typical dusky-gray respirator brain generally requires about 12 h of a nonperfused state (23,31). This time course is not influenced by delays in performance of the autopsy or ordinary delays in refrigeration of the body after death has been declared (23). The typical well-developed respirator brain shows considerable surface vasocongestion due to venous engorgement and sometimes thrombosis in cortical veins, the superior sagittal sinus and other venous outflow channels. Subarachnoid hemorrhage is common, even in cases where there is no obvious causal intracranial pathology to explain it. Its presence may be unrelated to the cause of death.

Coronal sectioning of the brain usually reveals congestion and overt intracortical hemorrhage (Fig. 3-3). This phenomenon is likely due to endothelial ischemia following excursions in cerebral perfusion, and reperfusion, leading to vascular damage and hemorrhage with possibly an element of venous infarction. The cortical hemorrhage and congestion is usually not uniform, but tends to be maximal in the end-perfusion territories of the major arterial supplies (watershed areas). The white matter is usually gray and soft and may contain perivascular hemorrhages. Again, it should be noted that nothing of a premortem causal nature can be inferred from white matter hemorrhages in any brain-dead specimen. The circulatory dysfunction inherent to the process will, by itself, produce petechial hemorrhages, effectively overwhelming any underlying lesion that might have arisen premortem. This may also include axonal balloons, thought by many to be the sine qua non of shear-force and rotational injury.

Some portions of the brain may remain relatively intact while substantial portions of the brain may display the typical respirator brain pathology (Fig. 3-4). In such cases electroencephalography may continue to demonstrate some electrocerebral activity and not isoelectric tracings (6).

With life support measures, the brain will generally remain relatively intact, though progressively soft, for about a week. Thereafter liquefaction evolves such that by two to three weeks the brain may be contained by the pia and immediate outer portion of the cortex. This part of the cortex can be nourished by diffusion from the meningeal circulation derived from external carotid blood flow. When an attempt is made to remove it at autopsy, however, it disintegrates. A serious problem for exam-

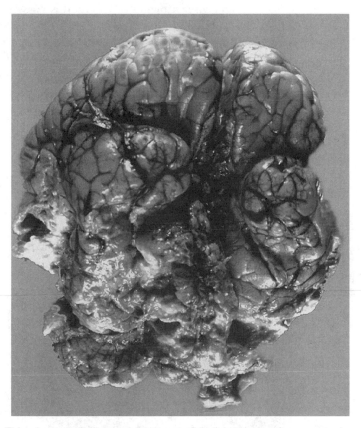

FIG. 3-4. This photograph illustrates that not all individuals on life support who eventually meet criteria for brain death have diffuse, uniform pathology. In this case, the brainstem, cerebellum, and more posterior parts of the brain are more liquefied than are the more anterior portions of the brain that were nourished by the internal carotid system. It is likely that individual variations in anatomy, possibly absence of one vertebral artery or minimal posterior communicating arteries, led to worse blood flow in these vascular territories than in those more anteriorly, leading to earlier necrosis and liquefaction. In such cases, there may be preservation of organized electrophysiological activity, rather than in cases where circulatory failure is more uniform.

ination is that respirator brains not only are fragile but also do not become more solid
upon formalin immersion. Due to autolysis, the protein cross-linking process of fixation by formalin or other fixatives cannot function because there are no intact proteins capable of being chemically cross linked. The progressive liquefaction of the
brain can result in a common artifact, now appreciated for what it is: sloughing of
necrotic cerebellar tissue into the subarachnoid space of the spinal cord. It is a very
common finding to discover autolytic or even relatively preserved cerebellar cortical
tissue surrounding the spinal cord (Fig. 3-5), usually in the subarachnoid space, but
also (microscopically) in the subdural space of the cord (32) (Fig. 3-6). It is not difficult to understand how cerebellar tissue could "drop" into the subarachnoid space
and be deposited at all levels of the spinal sac, but it is somewhat more problematic
how this tissue reaches the subdural compartment of the cord. It is possible that this
results from artifacts of sectioning and dissection, where essentially liquid material
is expressed by pressure of handling into the potential subdural spinal space.

Microscopically, the dead brain displays an exaggeration of artifacts of preparation that include pale or variable staining, bubbles, cracks, holes, and slits, and frag-

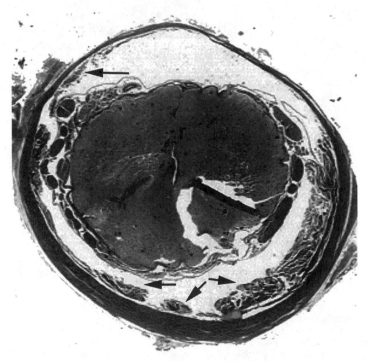

FIG. 3-5. This macrophotograph of the spinal cord and dura of a typical respirator brain in a child
abuse victim illustrates sloughed cerebellar cortical tissue (*arrows*) about the cord. It is not unusual to encounter large volumes of sloughed cortex about the cord, even to the level of the lum-
bar sac.

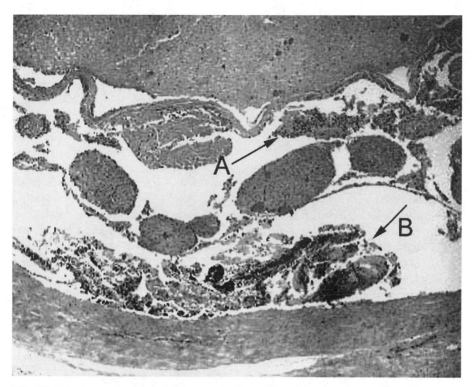

FIG. 3-6. The low-powered photomicrograph of a portion of the cord depicted in Figure 3-5 illustrates portions of the cord *(top)*, cross sections of nerve roots and the arachnoidal membrane approximated to them. Within the subarachnoid space *(arrow A)* there is sloughed cerebellar cortex. External to the arachnoid within the subdural "space" is much more sloughed cerebellum *(arrow B)* approximated to the dura *(below)*. It is not clear how this material came to rest in this location, but this is not an unusual microscopic finding.

mentation in the tissue. In the proper context of gross appearance and historical information these changes are consistent with a respirator brain but not necessarily diagnostic. These changes generally also do not provide reliable information on aging and dating of the processes. Since the evolutionary process of the respirator brain is ischemic and autolytic in nature, inflammation plays little role in the usual case. Unless there was a preceding infectious or inflammatory process in the brain, or inflammatory reaction to some other process, there will generally be little or absent inflammatory or scavenger cells in the meninges, or the brain. Occasionally, because of placement of intracranial pressure monitors, extraventricular drains or any other neurosurgical intervention, the intracranial compartment may become contaminated with bacteria. Bacteria may multiply unchecked but there is little or no circulatory mediated inflammatory response possible, except for a limited response via the meningeal circulation that is preserved through the external carotid circulation. This is a relatively uncommon phenomenon, and when observed has a subdued appearance over an inflammatory process in an intact brain. The microscopic abnormalities are summarized in Table 3-1.

There are many factors, largely poorly understood, that affect the temporal evolution of microscopic changes in the respirator brain. One of them is the underlying or preexisting health of the affected individual. Lindenberg (25,26) observed that the pathological expression of hypoxic-ischemic injury varied considerably between individuals who had been relatively acutely injured and those who were chronically ill. These differences were reflected in the time course and development of hypoxic-ischemic changes in neurons ("red" neurons) and the progression of autolytic changes in the brain with time.

Under ordinary circumstances, when an individual has been in a relatively functional and healthy state prior to brain death (e.g., due to acute myocardial failure, acute traumatic brain injury or subarachnoid hemorrhage), neurons damaged by one or a succession of ischemic-hypoxic insults may be irreversibly damaged but do not immediately display significant pathological changes. The first typical change is so-called "cloudy swelling" in which the neuron swells, and the cytoplasm loses some of its basophilia and distinctness. This phase is probably short-lived, to be replaced within an hour by a state commonly referred to as the red neuron (33–35). This change is manifested by the gradual eosinophilia of the cytoplasm of the neuron. It is accompanied by changes in the nucleus that consist of darkening, shrinkage with loss of detail and blurring in the chromatin and nucleolus, with eventual disappearance of the neuron. The topographic distribution of red neurons is that expected by individual location's vulnerability to hypoxia-ischemia, as outlined earlier.

The earliest appearance of red neurons is subject to debate. It has been claimed that this change is not manifest until about 8 to 12 h after the insult (36). Others suggest that red neurons can be observed earlier after hypoxic-ischemic insult (33), with red neurons in individuals who have survived as little as 2 h after an event (34,35). Examples of such circumstances involve documented intraoperative cardiovascular

TABLE 3-1. *Histopathology of brain death*

Site	Microscopy
Cortex	Almost invariably damaged; frank infarcts, congestion and edema; pink (hematoxylin and eosin) staining cytoplasm. No glial or hematogenous reaction.
Diencephalon	Periventricular edema; patchy, lytic changes in subthalamus, thalamus and hypothalamus (herniation effect).
Pituitary gland	May be spared (extracranial circulation; see Chapter 2). Petechial or confluent hemorrhages. Karyopyknotic changes in anterior lobe.
Brainstem	Flattened medulla oblongata, significant edema, hemorrhage, infarction and necrosis in mesencephalon but pons may be normal (15%).
Cerebellum	Swelling, congestion, fragmentation, granular layer is washed out due to lack of aniline dye stain. Purkinje cell layer is normal, edematous or devoid of all cells. Molecular layer is preserved.
Spinal cord	Normal, except upper cervical segments, dislocated cerebellar fragments.

From Walker AE. *Cerebral death,* 2nd ed. Baltimore: Urban & Schwarzenberg, 1981, with permission.

collapse, exsanguinations, or anesthetic accidents, drowning victims, and victims of strangulation or asphyxia. Some data on time course development of red neurons may be applicable from experimental studies and from *in vitro* preparations of animal brain (hippocampal slice studies), but how this applies to humans is conjectural. Unfortunately there has not been a systematic human study to determine the limits of detection, and how red neurons differ from patterns that are alleged to be due to artifact.

FORENSIC CONSIDERATIONS IN BRAIN DEATH

The neuropathologist may be able to offer important expertise that may aid in legal resolution of a case. A pervasive problem exists, however, when morphology and anatomy are called upon to determine functional status such as consciousness, awareness, cognition, and the ability to feel pain and experience suffering. These issues often become very fuzzy and may spark controversy amongst qualified experts. The most historically notorious forensic issue in connection with brain death is whether it can be declared with certainty.

A number of forensic issues have arisen in connection with continuation or withdrawal of life support in individuals who may have been the victim of criminal violence (see Chapter 8). A major issue, when it occurs, is that of possible "intervening cause" of death—the intervening cause possibly being the termination of life support. This situation may be reduced to the fundamental legal question (or assertion): who caused the death of the victim? The accused perpetrator or the physicians who terminated life support? An example of such case, described in more detail elsewhere (35), involved a quarrel between two lovers that culminated in a gunshot wound to the head. After some delay in seeking treatment, the wounded woman lapsed into unconsciousness. Someone in the medical team that attended her apparently regarded her as brain-dead and an organ salvage team supplanted normal medical care, leading eventually to organ salvage efforts and termination of life support rather than normal care, as would be expected for a gunshot wound to the head. The confusion that seemed to permeate this case was illustrated in the fact that there were multiple times and dates listed in the records of the declaration of death, the last being by the autopsy pathologist at the medical examiner's office. In this case, the defense attorneys for the man who shot the woman alleged that through the actions or rather inactions of the medical team and the apparent overriding issue of organ procurement, the victim died, suggesting an intervening cause of death of the victim.

A relatively common occurrence is the declaration of death or the policy of organ salvage in infants and children maintained on life support after possible child abuse. In such cases, the parents who may be the center of suspicion for having abused their child may be unwilling to permit removal of life support in the hope that "evidence" of their actions will remain obscure. On a practical note, even prolonged maintenance of a brain-dead child victim of potentially abusive head trauma on a respirator does not erase vital evidence of trauma or underlying disease processes, though it may make interpretation difficult.

It must be borne in mind that the intracranial circulation is totally nonfunctioning but the circulatory supply of the meninges (primarily dura) and the skull and pericranial tissues is intact since it is derived from supply of the external carotid artery. Thus, intracerebral processes become primarily necrotizing and retrogressive while exterior tissues are still capable of reacting with inflammatory responses, repair reactions and other vital processes. It is at the interface of these two systems, at the brain surface, subarachnoid space and meninges, where considerable variability of tissue reactions may occur, perhaps in an uneven or unpredictable manner—some mediated by direct circulation and others by diffusion. An important forensic issue, not yet resolved, is whether subdural hematomas age and evolve at the same rate no matter what the state of intracranial circulation is in. To the author's knowledge, no study has addressed this issue which may have considerable forensic importance in the arena of child abuse prosecution and defense.

Another subject is the diagnosis of diffuse axonal injury in the context of alleged child abuse fatality. The shaken baby syndrome varies in presentation from irritability to opisthotonus, seizures and coma. A full fontanelle and retinal hemorrhages are common but are not specific for diagnosis. Pathologic findings include fractures of posterior parietal or occipital bone, subdural hemorrhages (parieto-occipital and posterior interhemispheric fissure), superficial contusions in olfactory bulbs, gliding contusions, corpus callosum tears and diffuse axonal injury (37). According to many, diffuse axonal injury is a sine qua non of the so-called "shaken baby" syndrome and is, in fact, a definitive diagnostic marker for shaking trauma (38). Others have taken a more conservative view on this matter and have addressed a number of methodological flaws that question the reliability of the techniques employed and the interpretation of results (39–41). The process that many consider basic to the shaken baby syndrome is that, by vigorously and violently shaking a young infant, sufficient G forces and rotational shearing forces are generated within the brain to damage axons in many locations within the brain. These pathological changes may produce many of the symptoms of closed head injury observed in allegedly shaken babies such as immediate unconsciousness and cerebral edema. There are significant problems that surround the scientific veracity of this position; chief among them is biomechanical research that seems to show that simply shaking trauma alone cannot generate sufficient forces of any sort in the brain to produce the syndrome, and that to do so requires an impact (42). With an impact, even perhaps a comparatively "soft" one, the G forces with which the brain must cope are magnified 10 times or more. This is well within biomechanical parameters that have been shown by experiment (22,43) to produce axonal pathology and other injuries in animals.

Another not inconsequential material for thought involves interpretation of axonal pathology in postmortem specimens and the contribution of preexisting and accompanying processes such as hypoxia, ischemia, infarction, infection, edema, and herniation. All of these conditions can disturb the local axonal environments and physically disrupt effective axonal transport. Focal disruption produces axonal balloons and spheroids. The profound and multifocal circulatory disturbances that attend the evolving respirator brain may produce changes that might be impossible to differentiate from axonal injury caused by physical injury, particularly since a large percentage of allegedly abused babies need mechanical ventilation (44). Regrettably, the earlier studies on detection and interpretation of diffuse axonal injury in allegedly abused babies did not take these considerations into account in their controls (39,45). Furthermore, method of case selection may be important. It is rare that a caregiver will admit, let alone in sufficient detail, if shaking has occurred. Most published studies simply take the word of a committee or someone else that shaking occurred, and conclusions may be based on a biased primary selection variable.

This illustrates a compelling phenomenon: that of an examination of medical "facts" and conventions within the context of a nonmedical analytical exercise such as a civil or criminal trial. In this forum, it would not be unusual to engage in an in-depth examination of the scientific evidence or mechanism of disease as held by medical experts. This process is often very revealing to everyone, in that there may be complexities of great consequence in apparently simple conditions. However, the fund of knowledge that has been assumed may not be as robust as was thought (46).

REFERENCES

1. Cushing H. Some experimental and clinical observations concerning states of increased intracranial tension. *Am J Med Sci* 1902;124:375–400.
2. Mollaret P. Über die äussersten Möglichkeiten der Wiederbelebung: Die Grenzen zwischen Leben und Tod. München. *Med Wochenschr* 1962;104:1539–1545.
3. Kass LR. Death as an event: a community of Robert Morison. *Science* 1971;173:698–702.
4. Korein J. The problem of brain death: development and history. *Ann NY Acad Sci* 1978;315:6–18.
5. Collaborative Study. An appraisal of the criteria of cerebral death–a summary statement. *JAMA* 1977; 237:982–986.
6. Bennett DR, Hughes JR, Korein J, et al. *Atlas of electroencephalography in coma and cerebral death.* New York: Raven Press, 1976.
7. Walker AE. *Cerebral death,* 2nd ed. Baltimore: Urban & Schwarzenberg, 1981.
8. Marmarou A, Tabaddor K. Intracranial pressure: physiology and pathophysiology. In: Cooper PR, ed. *Head injury,* 3rd ed. Baltimore: Williams & Wilkins, 1993:203–224.
9. Feldman Z, Narayan RK. Intracranial pressure monitoring: techniques and pitfalls. In: Cooper PR, ed. *Head injury,* 3rd ed. Baltimore: Williams & Wilkins, 1993:247–274.
10. Chesnut RM. Treating raised intracranial pressure in head injury. In: Narayan RK, Wilberger Jr JE, Povlishock JT, eds. *Neurotrauma.* New York: McGraw-Hill, 1996:445–469.
11. Bakay RAE, Wood JH. Pathophysiology of cerebrospinal fluid in trauma. In: Becker DP, Povlishock JT, eds. *Central Nervous System Trauma Status Report 1985.* Washington, DC: National Institutes of Health, NINCDS, 1985:89–122.
12. Welch K. The principles of physiology of the cerebrospinal fluid in relation to hydrocephalus including normal pressure hydrocephalus. In: Friedlander WJ, ed. *Advances in neurology. Current reviews.* New York: Raven Press, 1975:345–375.
13. Welch K, Sadler K. Permeability of the choroid plexus of the rabbit to several solutes. *Am J Physiol* 1966;210:652–660.
14. Miller JD. Traumatic brain swelling and edema. In: Cooper PR, ed. *Head injury,* 3rd ed. Baltimore: Williams & Wilkins, 1993:331–354.
15. Bruce DA, Alavi A, Bilaniuk L, et al. Diffuse cerebral swelling following head injuries in children: the syndrome of "malignant brain edema." *J Neurosurg* 1981;54:170–178.
16. Snoek JW, Minderhous JM, Wilminik JT. Delayed deterioration following mild head injury in children. *Brain* 1984;107:15–36.
17. Muizelaar JP, Marmarou A, DeSalles AA, et al. Cerebral blood flow and metabolism in severely head-injured children. Part I: relationship with GCS, outcome, ICP and PVI. *J Neurosurg* 1989;71:63–71.
18. Muizelaar JP, Ward JD, Marmarou AM, et al. Cerebral blood flow in severely head-injured children. Part II: autoregulation. *J Neurosurg* 1989;71:72–76.

19. Sioutos PJ, Orozco JA, Carter LP. Regional cerebral blood flow techniques. In: Narayan RK, Wilberger Jr JE, Povlishock JT, eds. *Neurotrauma.* New York: McGraw-Hill, 1996:503–517.
20. Sokoloff L. Circulation and energy metabolism of the brain. In: Siegel GJ, Albers RW, Katzman R, Agranoff BW, eds. *Basic neurochemistry,* 2nd ed. Boston: Little, Brown, 1976:388–413.
21. Schade JP, McMenemey WH, eds. *Selective vulnerability of the brain in hypoxemia.* Oxford: Blackwell, 1963.
22. Gennarelli TA, Thibault LE, Adams JH, et al. Diffuse axonal injury and traumatic coma in the primate. *Ann Neurol* 1982;12:564–574.
23. Leestma JE, Hughes JR, Diamond ER. Temporal correlates in brain death. EEG and clinical relationships to the respirator brain. *Arch Neurol* 1984;41:147–152.
24. Hughes JR, Boshes B, Leestma JE. Electroclinical and pathologic correlations in comatose patients. *Clin Electroencephalogr* 1976;7:13–30.
25. Lindenberg RL. Anoxia does not produce brain damage. *Nippon Hoigaku Zasshi* 1981;36:38–57.
26. Lindenberg RL. Systemic oxygen deficiencies: the respirator brain. In: Mickler J, ed. *Pathology of the nervous system.* New York: McGraw-Hill, 1971:1583–1617.
27. Crone C. The blood–brain barrier: a modified tight epithelium. In: Suckling AJ, Rumsby MG, Bradbury MWB, eds. *The blood–brain barrier in health and disease.* Chichester, UK: Ellis Horwood, 1986:17–40.
28. Abbott NJ, Bundgaard M, Cserr HF. Comparative physiology of the blood–brain barrier. In: Suckling AJ, Rumsby MG, Gradbury MWB, eds. *Blood–brain barrier in health and disease.* Chichester, UK: Ellis Horwood, 1986:52–72.
29. Katzman R. Blood–brain–CSF barriers. In: Siegel GJ, Albers RW, Katzman R, Agranoff BW, eds. *Basic neurochemistry,* 2nd ed. Boston: Little, Brown, 1976:414–428.
30. Marmarou A. Pathophysiology of intracranial pressure. In: Narayan RK, Wilberger Jr JE, Povlishock JT, eds. *Neurotrauma.* New York: McGraw-Hill, 1996:413–428.
31. Leestma JE. Brain swelling and intracranial pressure effects. In: Leestma JE, ed. *Forensic neuropathology.* New York: Raven Press, 1988:157–183.
32. Herrick MK, Agamanolis DP. Displacement of cerebellar tissue into spinal canal. A component of the respirator brain syndrome. *Arch Pathol* 1975;99:565–571.
33. Garcia JH, Mena H. Vascular diseases. In: Garcia JH, ed. *Neuropathology: the diagnostic approach.* St. Louis: Mosby, 1997:263–320.
34. Leestma JE. Forensic aspects of general neuropathology. In: Leestma JE, ed. *Forensic neuropathology.* New York: Raven Press, 1988:24–156.
35. Leestma JE. Forensic neuropathology. In: Garcia JH, ed. *Neuropathology: the diagnostic approach.* St. Louis: Mosby, 1997:475–527.
36. Graham DI. Hypoxia and vascular disorders. In: Adams JH, Duchen LW, eds. *Greenfield's neuropathology,* 5th ed. New York: Oxford University Press, 1992:153–268.
37. Duhaime A-C, Christian CW, Rorke LB, et al. Nonaccidental head injury in infants—the shaken-baby syndrome. *N Engl J Med* 1998;338:1822–1829.
38. David TJ. Shaken baby (shaken impact) syndrome: non-accidental head injury in infancy. *J R Soc Med* 1999;92:556–561.
39. Gultekin SH, Smith TW. Diffuse axonal injury in craniocerebral trauma. A comparative histologic and immunohistochemical study. *Arch Pathol Lab Med* 1994;118:168–171.
40. Smith JW, Minderhous JM, Wilminik JT. Delayed deterioration following mild head injury in children. *Brain* 1984;107:15–36.
41. Shannon P, Smith CR, Deck J, et al. Axonal injury and the neuropathology of shaken baby syndrome. *Acta Neuropathol* 1998;95:625–631.
42. Duhaime A-C, Gennarelli TA, Thibault LE, et al. The shaken baby syndrome. A clinical, pathological, and biomechanical study. *J Neurosurg* 1987;66:409–415.
43. Gennarelli TA, Thibault LE. Biological models of head injury. In: Becker DP, Povlishock JT, eds. *Central Nervous System Trauma Status Report 1985.* Washington, DC: National Institutes of Health, NINCDS, 1985:391.
44. Oehmichen M, Meissner C, Schmidt V, et al. Axonal injury–a diagnostic tool in forensic neuropathology? A review. *Forensic Sci Int* 1998;95:67–83.
45. Vowles GH, Scholtz CL, Cameron JM. Diffuse axonal injury in early infancy. *J Clin Pathol* 1987;40:185–189.
46. Foster KR, Huber PW. *Judging science. Scientific knowledge and the Federal Courts.* Cambridge: MIT Press, 1997.

4

Clinical Diagnosis and Confirmatory Testing of Brain Death in Adults

Eelco F. M. Wijdicks

Department of Neurology, Mayo Clinic, Rochester, Minnesota

Brain death is anticipated in many cataclysmic neurologic disorders, but it represents only a small proportion of all medical and non–trauma-related surgical intensive care admissions. The incidence of brain death in specialized neurotrauma units is much higher, but again, a severely disabled functional state or death from cardiopulmonary arrest is a far more common outcome than loss of brain function. In our neurologic-neurosurgical intensive care unit, approximately 10 comatose patients per 1,000 acute admissions evolve into brain death. Compression, shift, and neuronal loss of diencephalic structures or brainstem due to an acute mass are common mechanisms, but a more diffuse anoxic-ischemic or overwhelming infection of the central nervous system may rapidly ravage both hemispheres. Precipitous loss of blood pressure and new-onset hypothermia or polyuria are the most characteristic clinical indicators that the brain has been completely destroyed.

This chapter discusses clinical assessment of brain death in adults. It expands on the American Academy of Neurology practice parameter document adopted in 1995 (1,2). A separate discussion concerning infants and children follows in Chapter 5. The determination of brain death in a person precious in the family's memory remains a painful task. Recommendations for family discussion and ways to advocate organ donation are found in Chapter 10.

CLINICAL EXAMINATION

Assessment of brain death in a comatose patient should proceed with a certain set of principles in mind, namely excluding major confounders, establishing the cause of the coma, ascertaining irreversibility, and accurately testing brainstem reflexes at all levels of the brainstem.

Clinical examination should proceed only if certain prerequisites are met (Table 4-1). In the vast majority of patients, computed tomography (CT) scanning shows a mass with herniation, multiple hemispheric lesions with edema, or edema alone. Obviously, a CT scan abnormality compatible with brain death does not obviate a search for confounders. Conversely, a normal CT scan can be seen early following cardiac or respiratory arrest and in patients with fulminant meningitis or encephalitis. In circumstances of overwhelming infection, examination of cerebrospinal fluid (CSF) should reveal diagnostic findings, such as pleocytosis, increased erythrocyte count, or positive Gram stain. Some viruses, parasites, and bacteria can be detected by poly-

TABLE 4-1. *Prerequisites before determination of brain death*

Definitive acute catastrophic event involving both hemispheres or brainstem and irreversibility
Exclusion of complicating medical conditions that may confound clinical assessment, particularly severe electrolyte, acid-base, or endocrine disturbances
Core temperature of ≥32°C
No documented evidence of drug intoxication, poisoning, or neuromuscular blocking agents

merase chain reaction (PCR), although not in due time. Interpretation of the CT scan in a patient suspected of being brain dead requires knowledge of the patterns that are compatible with brain death (Fig. 4-1). For example, in cases of traumatic brain injury, multiple contusions or a subdural or epidural hematoma should be present which displaces the septum pellucidum from its midline position. Effacement of the basal cistern and sulci is a common finding in patients with diffuse, profound cerebral edema. When major discrepancies exist between the clinical examination and the CT scan, a repeat CT study is warranted and often will document expansion of the mass or an enlarged mass effect. If the CT scan remains incongruent with loss of brain function, other factors should be considered, particularly drugs, poison, or an endocrine or major electrolyte abnormality. Core temperature should be at least 32°C. The potential consequences of these abnormalities for brain death determination are further elaborated on in Chapter 6. In any case, the clinical examination should be methodical and focus on (a) documentation of coma, (b) absence of brainstem reflexes, and (c) demonstration of apnea following maximal stimulation of respiratory centers after induction of acute CSF acidosis.

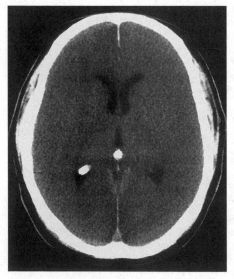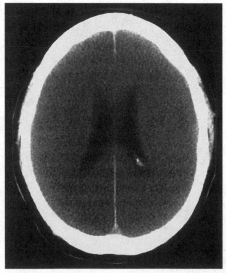

A   B

FIG. 4-1. Computed tomography scan patterns commonly seen in patients at time of brain death determination. **A,B:** Cerebral edema following cardiac or respiratory arrest. Note featureless brain with absent sulci and no white matter–gray matter differentiation. *(continued)*

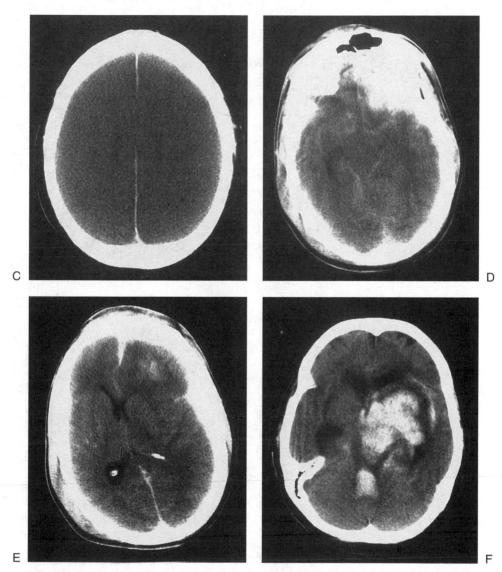

FIG. 4-1. *Continued.* **C:** Cerebral edema following cardiac or respiratory arrest. Note featureless brain with absent sulci and no white matter–gray matter differentiation. **D,E:** Left subdural hematoma and frontal contusion with pronounced shift of the midline structures and septum pellucidum. Early enlargement of the temporal horn and effacement of basal cisterns are seen. **F:** Destructive hemorrhage into the putamen with thalamus extension and hemoventricle. *(continued)*

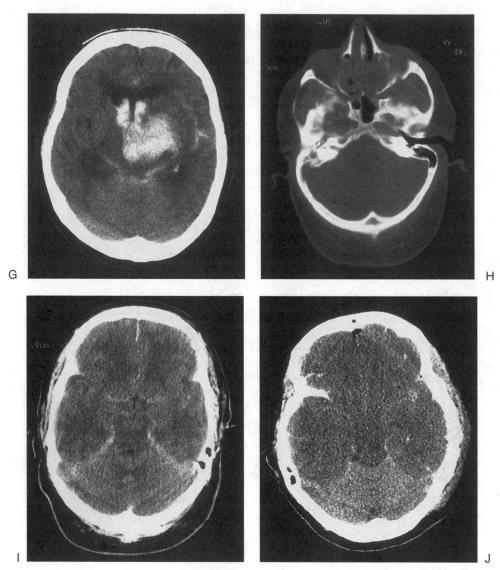

FIG. 4-1. *Continued.* **G:** Destructive putamen hemorrhage with thalamus extension and hemoventricle. **H,I:** Cerebral edema in patient with fulminant pneumococcal meningitis. Note opacification of the right mastoid air cells due to inflammatory disease. *(continued).*

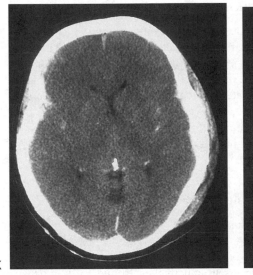
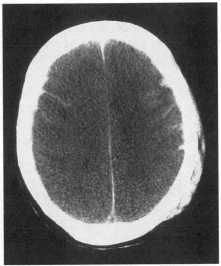

K   L

FIG. 4-1. *Continued.* **J–L:** Traumatic brain edema with multiple contusions.

Coma

Patients lack all evidence of responsiveness due to complete loss of consciousness.

Technique

The depth of coma can be assessed by examining eye and motor responses with the use of standard painful stimuli such as pressure on the supraorbital nerve, nail bed pressure, and temporomandibular joint compression (3). Other pain stimuli, such as sternal rubbing, rubbing knuckles against the ribs in the axilla, twisting the forearm or nipples, and applying pin prick on several body locations, may be equally effective but have not been accepted as the norm. Eye opening and motor responses to voice or pain should be absent on repeated tests (Fig. 4-2).

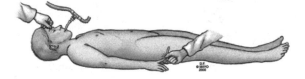

FIG. 4-2. Motor response to pain. (By permission of Mayo Foundation.)

Alerts

Motor responses may occur spontaneously, after painful stimulation, and during apnea testing, particularly when hypoxemia or hypotension intervenes. These responses should be interpreted as spinally generated. They are brief, slow movements in the upper limbs, flexion in the fingers, or arm lifting, and they do not become integrated into truly coordinated decerebrate or decorticate responses. They seldom persist with repeated stimulation. Reproducible eye opening, but with only a minimal eyelid elevation barely showing the beginning of an iris, has been noted in response to twisting of a nipple in patients who fulfilled all clinical criteria of brain death (4,5). The reflex pathway is not known.

Absence of Brainstem Reflexes

Examination of Pupils

Technique

The response to bright light should be absent in both eyes. Round, oval, or irregularly shaped pupils are compatible with brain death. Most pupils in brain death are in mid position (4 to 6 mm) (6). Dilated pupils are compatible with brain death because intact sympathetic cervical spine pathways connected to the radially arranged fibers of the dilator muscle may remain intact (Fig. 4-3).

Alerts

Many drugs can influence pupil size, but the light response remains intact. In conventional doses, atropine given intravenously has no marked influence on the pupillary response (7,8). Short-term neuromuscular blocking drugs do not noticeably in-

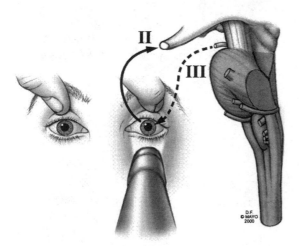

FIG. 4-3. Pupil size and light response. Roman numerals refer to cranial nerves. (By permission of Mayo Foundation.)

fluence pupil size (9), but a recent report with escalating doses of atracurium and vecuronium documented reversible mydriasis and ultimately nonreactive light responses (10). Topical ocular instillation of drugs and trauma to the cornea or bulbus oculi may cause abnormalities in pupil size and can produce nonreactive pupils. Preexisting anatomic abnormalities of the iris or effects of previous surgery should be excluded.

Examination of Ocular Movements

Technique

Ocular movements should be absent, including any type of nystagmus. The oculocephalic reflex, elicited by fast turning of the head from middle position to 90 degrees on both sides, may not be sensitive enough to document the absence of ocular movements.

Ocular movements are also absent after caloric testing with ice water. Caloric testing should preferably be done with the head elevated to 30 degrees during irrigation of the tympanum on each side. With 30 degrees elevation, the horizontal canal becomes vertical. Irrigation of the tympanum can best be accomplished by inserting a small suction catheter into the external auditory canal and connecting it to a 50-mL syringe filled with ice water. A cold stimulus results in sedimentation of the endolymph and stimulation of the hair cells. The normal response in a comatose patient is a slow deviation of the eyes directed to the cold caloric stimulus. The response is absent in brain death. Absent eye movement may be very difficult to appreciate, and placement of pen marks on the lower eyelid at the level of the pupil may be helpful. One should allow up to 1 min of observation after injection, and the time between stimulation on each side should be at least 5 min, to reduce a possible overriding effect from the opposite irrigated ear (Fig. 4-4).

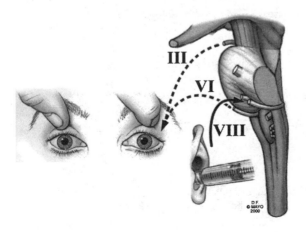

FIG. 4-4. Caloric testing. Roman numerals refer to cranial nerves. (By permission of Mayo Foundation.)

Alerts

Clotted blood or cerumen in the ear may diminish the caloric response, and repeat testing is required. It is prudent to inspect the tympanum directly and to document free access to the cold water injection. Presence of a ruptured eardrum will enhance the caloric response, but such a maneuver can only be allowed when brain death is highly probable. Prior exposure to toxic levels of certain drugs can diminish or completely abolish the caloric response. Some typical examples are aminoglycosides, tricyclic antidepressants, anticholinergics, antiepileptic drugs, and chemotherapeutic agents, among others (11). After closed head injury or facial trauma, eyelid edema and chemosis of the conjunctiva may limit movement of the globes. Basal fracture of the petrous bone abolishes the caloric response only unilaterally and may be identified by the presence of an ecchymotic mastoid process (Battle's sign).

Examination of Facial Sensation and Facial Motor Response

Technique

Absent corneal reflexes should be confirmed with a throat swab. Blinking requires intact brainstem reflex pathways and is not compatible with brain death. Facial myokymias could be due to muscle contraction from denervation or deafferentation of the facial nucleus and thus are compatible with brain death. Absent grimacing to pain can be documented by applying deep pressure with a blunt object on the nail beds, pressure on the supraorbital nerve, or deep pressure on both condyles at the level of the temporomandibular joint (Fig. 4-5). The jaw reflex should also be absent.

Alerts

Severe facial and ocular trauma may limit or eliminate interpretation of these brainstem reflexes.

Examination of Pharyngeal and Tracheal Reflexes

Technique

Lack of a cough response to bronchial suctioning should be demonstrated by passing a catheter through the endotracheal tube and providing suctioning pressure for several seconds (Fig. 4-6). Although not required as a test, 2 mg of atropine will not produce tachycardia. No change in heart rate after suctioning or atropine is further confirmatory of destruction of the intracranial parasympathetic pathways.

Alerts

In orally intubated patients, the gag response may be difficult to interpret and likely unreliable.

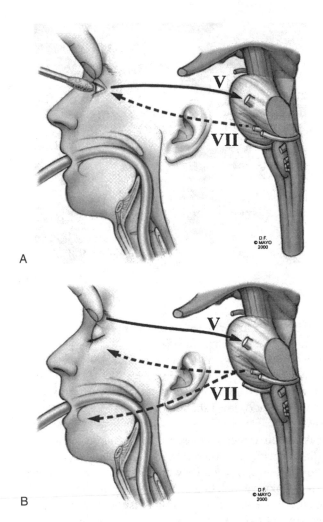

FIG. 4-5. Corneal reflex **(A)** and facial response to pain pressure on the supraorbital nerve **(B)**. Roman numerals refer to cranial nerves. (By permission of Mayo Foundation.)

Apnea

Apneic oxygenation is the most commonly used technique to demonstrate lack of ventilatory drive. This diagnostic tool involves placement of a source of 100% oxygen in the trachea which, through convection, results in oxygen flowing into the lungs (12–15). Preoxygenation eliminates the nitrogen stores in the respiratory tract and thus facilitates oxygen transport. On the basis of animal experiments and clinical observations, a target $PaCO_2$ of 60 mm Hg has been proposed as a level at which the medullary respiratory centers are maximally stimulated. Traditionally, it has been assumed that the respiratory centers are reset higher due to malfunction from brainstem

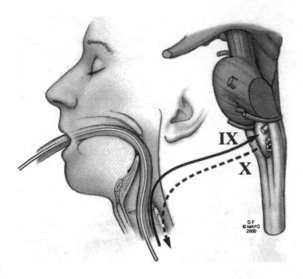

FIG. 4-6. Cough response. Roman numerals refer to cranial nerves. (By permission of Mayo Foundation.)

injury. The target, however, may be much lower, because in the few patients who started to breathe after disconnection of the ventilator, $Paco_2$ levels were in the low 30's. We have personally seen two patients who started to breathe at $Paco_2$ levels around 35 mm Hg but lost respiratory drive hours later. However, without detailed documentation on large numbers of patients, a $Paco_2$ increase to 60 mm Hg or a 20 mm Hg increase from a normal baseline $Paco_2$ level should remain the recommended target (for an historical overview, see Chapter 1).

The increase in $Paco_2$ is biphasic, with a steep increase in the first minutes due to equilibration of arterial carbon dioxide with mixed central venous carbon dioxide. In the tracheobronchial phase of the apnea test, oxygen flow ensures uptake of oxygen in pulmonary capillaries, but carbon dioxide exhalation does not take place and therefore there is a rapid rise of $Paco_2$ due to metabolic production of carbon dioxide. Increase in $Paco_2$ results in a decrease in CSF pH, which is sensed by the medullary respiratory centers and, when function is present, results in a respiratory drive (16,17). A rapid increase in $Paco_2$ to 60 mm Hg or 20 mm Hg above normal baseline maximally stimulates these centers, also because CSF is unable to buffer acidosis with blood bicarbonate owing to its slower diffusion than carbon dioxide.

Many physicians prefer simple disconnection of the ventilator and use of oxygen flow through an endotracheally placed catheter. In addition to monitoring of oxygen saturation, pulse, and blood pressure, visual inspection of thoracic and abdominal movement is required. Disconnecting the patient from the ventilator reduces artifact reading of breathing on the ventilator display often due to continuous positive airway pressure (CPAP) alone. We have noted significant false readings (spontaneous respiratory rates of 20 to 30 per minute) by mechanical ventilator sensors with settings as low as a CPAP of 2.

Lang (18) has suggested a possibly attractive method of carbon dioxide augmentation to reduce observation time, but an overshoot to potentially dangerous hypercarbia is a concern. Monitoring carbon dioxide by using a transcutaneous device may reduce carbon dioxide target overshoot, but discrepancies between transcutaneous and arterial carbon dioxide may be substantial.

Alternatively, manipulating $Paco_2$ upward by using hypoventilation with end-tidal carbon dioxide monitoring devices has been suggested as a method. It can be cumbersome not only because of the inability to predict $Paco_2$ but also because the method may lead to gradual CSF buffering and thus failure to produce acute acidosis in the CSF compartment.

Testing for apnea in a patient with otherwise absent brainstem reflexes is standard, and a positive test (no breathing with target $Paco_2$) confirms brain death. The procedure, however, has generated some debate. The arguments against the apnea test are as follows. First, in the event of preserved respiration, the outcome is similar. No report has been published of an adult patient who, with otherwise absent brainstem reflexes but spontaneous breathing, "recovers" to a persistent vegetative state or better. Second, the procedure may induce hypotension and hypoxemia, which potentially may render organs unsuitable for transplantation. There are no data in the transplant literature to support this contention (19–21). The apnea test may be very difficult to perform (e.g., because of preservation of adequate oxygenation) in patients with marginal lung function due to contusion or pulmonary edema. Some have argued, and incorrectly so, that hypoxemia or acidosis will result in death of some viable neurons and thus cause brain death. It is one of the reasons behind the Japanese criteria of performing an EEG before an apnea test (see Chapter 1). We believe the apnea test is essential because prolonged preserved medulla oblongata function may occur (see Chapter 6) and its presence can only be detected by a formal apnea test.

The apnea test is generally safe with careful precautions. First, hypothermia should be corrected from $32°C$ (prerequisite for determination of brain death) to normothermia ($36°C$ to $37°C$). In hypothermia, carbon dioxide production may be delayed because of decreased metabolism. Moreover, in hypothermia the oxyhemoglobin dissociation curve shifts to the left, resulting in a decreased oxygen release. Second, persistent hypotension should be corrected and often requires a bolus of 5% albumin or an increase in administration of intravenous dopamine. The presence of a blood pressure of 90 to 100 mm Hg is probably acceptable before an apnea test. Other precautions are shown in Figure 4-7. If one holds to these strict guidelines, the apnea test is generally safe (22).

At the start of the apnea test, a $Paco_2$ within the normal range (35 to 45 mm Hg) is preferred. One can expect the $Paco_2$ to increase 3 to 6 mm Hg per minute (23). Therefore, when the $Paco_2$ is in the normal range, 8 min of disconnection should be sufficient to reach the target level of 60 mm Hg or to produce an increase of 20 mm Hg (Fig. 4-7) (24–27). Apnea can be confirmed with skin sensors from the electrocardiogram leads. On the monitor, these sensors should show only a cardiac artifact and no displacement indicating a breathing effort. Visual inspection of the rib cage and

P R E C A U T I O N S

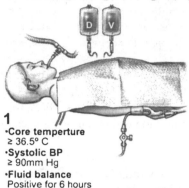

1
•**Core temperture**
≥ 36.5° C
•**Systolic BP**
≥ 90mm Hg
•**Fluid balance**
Positive for 6 hours

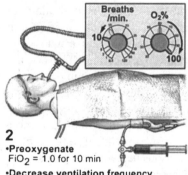

2
•**Preoxygenate**
FiO$_2$ = 1.0 for 10 min

•**Decrease ventilation frequency**
10 breaths/min (Tidal volume 10 ml/kg)

•**Arterial blood gas**
PO$_2$ ≥ 200mm Hg
PCO$_2$ ≥ 40mm Hg

P R O C E D U R E

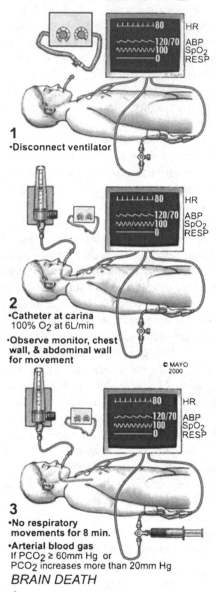

1
•**Disconnect ventilator**

2
•**Catheter at carina**
100% O$_2$ at 6L/min

•**Observe monitor, chest
wall, & abdominal wall
for movement**

© MAYO
2000

3
•**No respiratory
movements for 8 min.**
•**Arterial blood gas**
If PCO$_2$ ≥ 60mm Hg or
PCO$_2$ increases more than 20mm Hg

BRAIN DEATH

4
•**Reconnect ventilator** 10 breaths/min.

abdomen typically may show minimal movement synchronous with the heartbeat, less frequently some shoulder elevation, and intercostal retraction in the upper thorax.

Hypotension is the most common complication of the apnea test (22,28–30), and the patient should be reconnected to the ventilator when the blood pressure drops precipitously to 70 mm Hg systolic. Failure to preoxygenate remains an important cause of hypotension during apnea testing. However, when normal oxygen saturation is present, the induced acidosis may reduce myocardial contractility, usually when pH reaches 7.2. Moderate hypercapnia associated with respiratory acidosis does not induce ventricular dysfunction as measured by transesophageal echocardiography (31). Hypotension without hypoxemia during the apnea test often indicates that the $Paco_2$ has amply passed 60 mm Hg. Cardiac arrest from the procedure is exceedingly rare; we noted one instance in 145 consecutive procedures (22). Again, cardiac arrhythmias generally occur in patients whose hypoxemia is not corrected with oxygen supplementation during the apnea test. Patients who have had cardiac arrhythmias during the evolution of the neurologic catastrophe may not have them during the apnea test, and their presence should not preclude apnea testing. When hypoxemia occurs despite adequate preoxygenation and oxygen supply, al Jumah et al. (13) suggested performing the apnea test with the patient connected with zero rate, zero CPAP Fio_2 of 1.0, and continuous flow of 40 L/min (15 L/min for pediatric patients; bulk diffusion apnea test). It may still not be an alternative in patients with severe underlying pulmonary disease (13). Failure to adequately perform the apnea test should be followed by a confirmatory test if organ donation is considered.

SPINAL ACTIVITY

Body movements after death have been observed, generally during the apnea test but also during nurse preparation for transport, at the time of abdominal incision for organ retrieval, and in the morgue itself. As early as 1971, Goulon et al. (32) supplemented their original paper with additional descriptions of body movements brought on by light stimulation–triple retreat of the legs, adduction or abduction of the arm to

---

FIG. 4-7. Performance of the apnea test. The apnea test should be optimized by precautionary measures *(left)*. 1. Increasing core temperature to reduce possible effect of hypothermia on CO_2 production; reducing chances of hypotension by stabilizing blood pressure and hemodynamic state. 2. Preoxygenation aiming at Po_2 of at least 200 mm Hg, correcting possible hypocapnea (often due to hyperventilation; caused by high tidal volumes of the mechanical ventilator or possibly due to hypothermia). The apnea test can proceed as follows *(right)*. 1. Disconnect the ventilator while monitoring heart rate and blood pressure and possible respiratory excursions. 2. Provide adequate oxygen source, preferably with a catheter at the carina. 3. If no respiratory movements are observed, draw new blood gas. If Pco_2 rise fulfills criteria, reconnect ventilator. Any drop in blood pressure (BP ≤ 70 mm Hg) or cardiac arrhythmia should prompt the physician to abort the procedure and perform a confirmatory test (EEG, TCD, cerebral blood flow study). ABP, arterial blood pressure; BP, blood pressure; D, dopamine; HR, heart rate; RESP, respirations; Spo2, oxygen saturation by pulse oximetry; V, vasopressin. (By permission of Mayo Foundation.)

the stimulated area, and head rotation. These movements have puzzled the mind and have frightened family members. Evidence that the movements represent only spinal activity is the consistent clinical documentation of brain death with confirmation by an isoelectric electroencephalogram or the absence of intracranial flow. The most impressive body movement is a brief attempt of the body to sit up to 40 to 60 degrees but generally not in a full sitting position. Arms may be raised independently of each other; legs seldom move. Rhythmic flexion of the hip and knee mimicking stepping has occurred at the pontomedullary stage of herniation, but it disappears in brain death (33). These are slow movements, lasting 10 to 20 s. A painful stimulus rarely produces these complex movements, but we and others have observed them after forceful flexion of the neck or rotation of the body (e.g., when replacing bed linen; Fig. 4-8). A videotape has recently become available (34). Head turning consistently to one side (35) and back arching may occur. Sometimes a body may partly roll over and dislodge catheters (36,37). These movements have been named "Lazarus signs," referring to the biblical person said to have been raised by Jesus, but the term is disrespectful to the patient or family and should be avoided in conversation.

Some of this spinal activity may be triggered by the ventilator, synchronous with pulmonary insufflation (38), and disappear after disconnection of the ventilator. A recent prospective study of 38 patients with brain death, mostly young adults, found a surprisingly high frequency of spinal-generated movements (39%), but included a triple flexion response, facial myokymias, and finger jerks (36).

Other manifestations include the undulating toe sign (snapping the big toe leads to an undulating movement of the toes resembling those of a sea anemone) (39), persistent Babinski response, any tendon, abdominal, or cremaster reflex, flushing, shivering, sweating, and myoclonic twitching in limb muscles. The most commonly observed reflexes and movements are shown in Table 4-2. Usually these movements are single events, but if they are recurrent, paralytic agents should be used to prevent them during organ retrieval.

PRIMARY BRAINSTEM DEATH

Acute neurologic injury may be confined to the brainstem, but is very uncommon. In many destructive lesions of the brainstem (e.g., ruptured basilar aneurysm), secondary damage to the hemispheres from ischemic injury may have intervened. Conditions associated with isolated brainstem death include pontine hemorrhage, basilar artery embolus, and, not uncommonly, gunshot wounds due to a suicide attempt, especially when the barrel of the gun has been placed inside the mouth. The brain hemispheres remain initially untouched until massive hydrocephalus increases intracranial pressure and impedes intracranial flow. This condition is akin to "cerveau isolé." Mature cats with the entire brainstem and cerebellum removed displayed EEG activity with commonly observed sleep spindles (40). A confirmation test will only confuse the matter, because cerebral blood flow is likely to be present, particularly when the test is performed early. Electroencephalography may show nonreactive alpha or

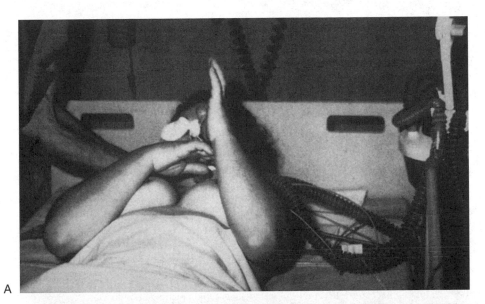

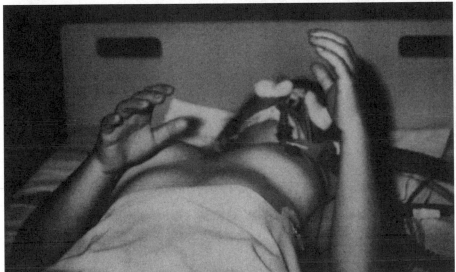

FIG. 4-8. Arm elevation with neck flexion **(A)** and spontaneously **(B)**. (From Turmel A, Roux A, Bojanowski MW. Spinal man after declaration of brain death. *Neurosurgery* 1991;28:298–302, with permission of the Congress of Neurological Surgeons.)

TABLE 4-2. *Spinal movements and reflexes in brain death*

Cervical spine
  Tonic neck reflexes (neck flexion)
    Neck-abdominal muscle contraction
    Neck-hip flexion
    Neck-arm flexion
    Neck-shoulder protrusion
  Head turning to side
Upper extremity
  Flexion-withdrawal reflex
  Unilateral extension-pronation
  Isolated finger jerks; finger pinch-finger flexion
  Flexion elevation of arm; joining of hands possible
Trunk
  Asymmetric opisthotonic posturing of trunk
  Flexion of trunk, causing partial sitting movements
  Abdominal reflexes
Lower extremity
  Plantar flexion of toes after percussion
  Triple flexion, Babinski sign

From Goulon M, Nouailhat F, Babinet P. Irreversible coma [French]. *Ann Med Interne* 1971;122:479–486; Hanna JP, Frank JI. Automatic stepping in the pontomedullary stage of central herniation. *Neurology* 1995;45:985–986; Bueri JA, Saposnik G, Maurino J, et al. Lazarus' sign in brain death. *Movement Disorders* 2000;15:583–586; Christie JM, O'Lenic TD, Cane RD. Head turning in brain death. *J Clin Anesth* 1996;8:141–143; Saposnik G, Bueri JA, Maurino J et al. Spontaneous and reflex movements in brain death. *Neurology* 2000;54:221–223; Ropper AH. Unusual spontaneous movements in brain-dead patients. *Neurology* 1984;34:1089–1092; Martí-Fàbregas J, López-Navidad A, Caballero F, et al. Decerebrate-like posturing with mechanical ventilation in brain death. *Neurology* 2000;54:224–227; and Fujimoto K, Yamauchi Y, Yoshida M. Spinal myoclonus in association with brain death [Japanese]. *Rinsho ShinKeigaku* 1989;29:1417–1419.

spindle coma patterns. A possible approach is to extend observation time to 24 h, followed by a full repeat neurologic examination (including apnea test). A confirmation test can be considered after this period of long observation but should not be mandatory. In the United States, primary brainstem death does not fit into the concept of whole brain death, but it has been accepted in the United Kingdom and rightly so, because no survivor has been reported when all brainstem function has been lost.

OBSERVATION PERIOD

A reasonable effort should be made to allow an observation period after the clinical criteria of brain death have been met. The American Academy of Neurology practice parameters optionally call for 6 h of observation and repeat testing. This is a long way from the original 24-h observation, and Cantu's statement of nearly 30 years ago still carries some truth:

Today, many potential donor organs are lost from patients with irreversible brain damage because of the required waiting-period of at least 24 h to obtain two flat EEGs. The waiting-period is often longer than 24 h if EEGs are not readily available. The importance of this loss is brought into perspective when we realise that there are now 70 people on dialysis awaiting cadaver-kidney transplantation at one major Boston hospital alone (41).

Repeat examination should include all brainstem reflexes, but it is not necessary to repeat a formal apnea test. No adult patient is on record in whom breathing resumed after initial adequate documentation of apnea. Many patients may have started to develop labile blood pressure and early neurogenic pulmonary edema, and the observation period can certainly be shortened if a recipient is waiting or when a confirmatory laboratory test has been performed.

PHYSICIAN COMPETENCY IN BRAIN DEATH DETERMINATION

At first sight, it is correctly asserted that the determination of brain death is difficult. Nothing illustrates the complexity of this assessment better than the persistent reports of blatant errors in judgment not only in the medical literature but also in the lay press and on the Internet (42,43). Unfortunately, even gross misjudgments surface in the neurologic literature (44). As mentioned, determination of brain death requires not only the proper execution of a series of neurologic tests but also resolution of misleading clinical signs, interpretation of neuroimaging studies, interpretation of possible confounding factors, and determination of a need for confirmatory laboratory tests. Neurologists are often not available on a timely basis, particularly in rural areas. Naturally, any physician should be able to diagnose brain death, but a careful neurologic evaluation requires experience. The clinical examination of patients who are presumed brain dead should be academically precise and fully documented. To avoid any potential conflict, it is common practice to exclude transplant surgeons who are involved in prospective recovery of organs from performing examinations. No one in our practice finds this exclusion denigrating. There are no data to suggest that a second assessment by a different physician reduces errors or avoids neglect of key elements of the neurologic examination. Surprisingly, some states and a large number of hospitals in the United States continue to insist on a second independent examination. This approach not only may delay a declaration of death and thereby potentially jeopardize harvesting of vital organs (as hemodynamic instability and neurogenic pulmonary edema progress) but also may result in examination of a brain-dead patient by a less experienced physician urgently called upon. Even more surprisingly, in Virginia the brain death statute requires that a specialist in the neurosciences make the assessment (see Chapter 8).

So, who does qualify, and are determinations of brain death up to the mark? No formal audits of neurologists and neurosurgeons have been performed recently, but there is no reason to question competence. In our experience with many hundreds of brain death determinations performed by neurologists and neurosurgeons, grossly incomplete examinations were exceptional. Interpretation of unexpected findings, such as retained spinal reflex movements, could lead to a debate but was easily resolved. Intensive care neurologists and neurosurgeons are eminently qualified, but anesthesiologists and medical or surgical intensivists should be considered if they have maintained their clinical skills (42). A separate team or service would be ideal and would minimize errors and facilitate communication with transplant surgeons and donation agencies. Development of special certificates, as in resuscitation medicine, may need serious consideration.

CONFIRMATORY TEST IN ADULTS WITH BRAIN DEATH

Cerebral angiography, electroencephalography, transcranial ultrasonography, and a radionuclide scan can confirm the clinical diagnosis of brain death. Confirmatory tests are recommended in children less than 1 year old and in the occasional situation in which components of clinical testing cannot be reliably evaluated. In several European and Asiatic countries, confirmatory testing is mandated by law. It may be a contradiction of our time not to rely entirely on technologic devices to confirm brain death, but these tests should be performed only to confirm the clinical examination. The ideal practice is to use confirmatory tests after the neurologic examination has unequivocally shown that the patient no longer has any brain function.

Unfortunately, situations arise in which a confirmatory test has been performed before the formal clinical evaluation for possible brain death. In certain circumstances, a confirmatory test may show the presence of blood flow or electroencephalographic activity despite the absence of all brainstem function. This occurs in patients who had their confirmatory tests very early in the determination of brain death and particularly in those in whom the mechanism was other than increased intracranial pressure. It is appropriate not to rely on technical confirmatory tests when they are at odds with a clinical neurologic examination. Confirmatory tests in adults are described in this section, but details are also found in the chapter on brain death in children, where they are more relevant.

A recent disturbing study from Barcelona (45) suggested transcranial Doppler or nuclear scan to "speed up" the diagnosis of brain death in patients with recent administration of barbiturates, benzodiazepines, or opiates. This practice should be strongly rejected. Physicians should not go so far as to place blind faith in machinery and the clinical diagnosis remains a sacrosanct principle.

Cerebral Angiogram

A cerebral angiogram using the Seldinger technique through femoral arteries should document nonfilling of intracranial arteries (41,46–53). Increased intracranial pressure leads to increased cerebral vascular resistance, extreme slowing of flow, and circulatory arrest (54). Perivascular glial swelling and subintimal bleb formation from ischemia collapse the smaller vessels, leading to increased cerebrovascular resistance, but another mechanism of absent intracranial flow is destruction of the intracerebral vascular tree in conjunction with necrosis of the brain. The common carotid artery commonly bifurcates at C3–C4 into the internal and external portions.

The carotid bifurcation to the skull base is called the cervical segment until it enters the carotid canal. The petrous segment ascends 1 cm, then becomes horizontal until it enters the intracranial space at the foramen lacerum. The carotid artery then continues as the cavernous segment. The vertebral artery pierces the dura after traversing the atlanto-occipital membrane and this transition can at times be seen as a smooth band on a normal film. The carotid circulation will demonstrate circulatory arrest first, but the vertebral circulation can still show filling. This can be due to a supratentorial mass that has not transferred pressure to the posterior fossa resulting in cerebellar tonsillar herniation.

Contrast is injected under high pressure in both the anterior and the posterior circulation. With current standardized injection force, it is unlikely that flow can be artificially created by increasing injection pressure. Normally, the intracranial arteries fill first (low-resistance system), followed by the external arteries (high-resistance system). This is reversed with cerebral death. Arch aortography with lateral and anteroposterior views will show the contrast column in the carotids usually arresting abruptly at the level of the skull base at the petrous region of the internal carotid arteries. It should not fill the siphon. The vertebral system will opacify from the aortic arch injection, and a selective vertebral artery injection is not needed. The dye column in the vertebral artery arrests at the atlanto-occipital junction and the contrast level may reach C1 to C2 in 50% of patients. The external carotid circulation remains patent and fills rapidly and early, as opposed to slow filling of the remaining portion of the carotid circulation (Fig. 4-9). Delayed visualization of the superior sagittal sinus results from perfusion through meningeal vessels from the external carotid artery supply or from emissary veins. Some protocols consider at least two injections of contrast medium given with an interval of 20 min to establish persistent absent flow to the brain and thus total neuronal necrosis. Criteria for confirmation of brain death using cerebral angiography have not been developed by neuroradiologic societies.

Electroencephalography

Electroencephalography (EEG) has been used in the determination of brain death in many countries, and it remains an important confirmatory test (55–60). Usually, a 16- or 18-channel instrument is used, and recordings are obtained for at least 30 min. Typically, electrical activity is absent above 2 μV at a sensitivity of 2 μV/mm with a filter setting at 0.1 or 0.3 s and 70 Hz (61). There are, however, several examples of abnormal but existing EEG activity that may continue for several hours to days. In one consecutive study of patients who fulfilled the clinical criteria of brain death, 20% of 56 patients had residual EEG activity that lasted up to 168 h. In general, the sensitivity as well as the specificity of EEG is 90% (62). It should be noted that artifacts are common if a high gain amplification is used in an intensive care environment, with a significant possibility for electrical artifacts. EEG is used in many countries throughout the world, and because of its wide availability it remains a preferred confirmatory test (Fig. 4-10).

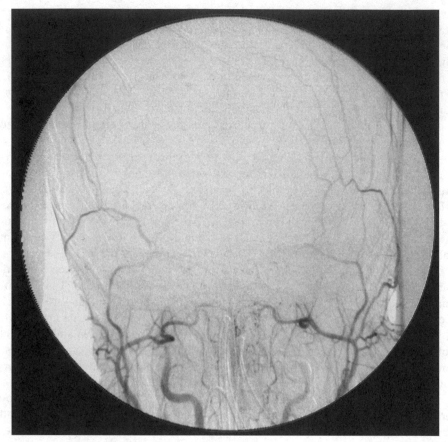

FIG. 4-9. Cerebral angiogram. Arch injection showing absent intracranial flow. The intracranial arteries are not identified, and the vertebral arteries stop below the skull base at C1–C2. Arterial filling involves only the external carotid branches.

Transcranial Doppler Sonography

Transcranial Doppler (TCD) is a validated confirmatory test, with sensitivity varying from 91% to 99% and a specificity of 100% (63–74). A portable Doppler device is used with insonating of both middle cerebral arteries through the temporal bone

FIG. 4-10. A: Isoelectric electroencephalogram (EEG) using standard recordings with high-sensitivity artifact is seen from a poorly filled electrode and pulse artifact. **B:** Electroretinogram is typically seen with photic stimulation in the frontal leads due to high sensitivity. It is eliminated with covering of each eye. For recommendations for recording electroencephalogram in cases of brain death, see text. **C:** EEG with electrocardiographic artifact. (By permission of the Massachusetts Medical Society.)

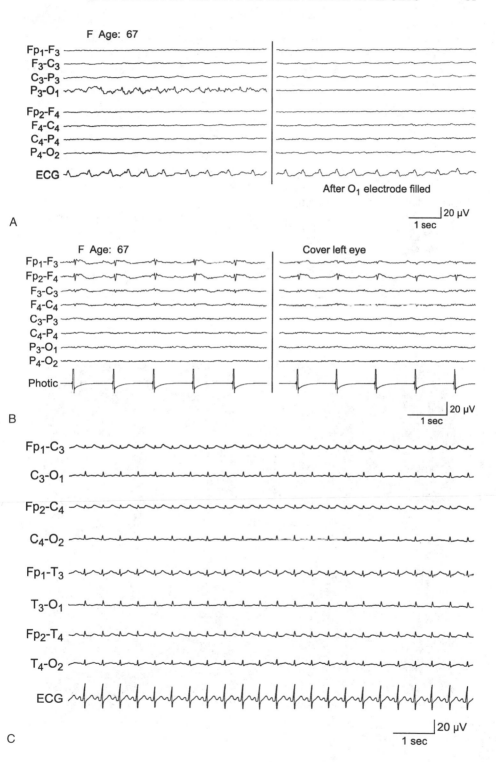

above the zygomatic arch. Absent flow intracranially may be due to transmission difficulties and in itself is not a criterion for brain death. In brain death, the typical transcranial Doppler signals, produced by the contractive forces of the arteries, are oscillating flow, defined by signals with forward and reverse flow components in one cardiac cycle (72). Most of the time, small (less than 50 cm/s) peaks in early systole, indicating very high vascular resistance, are recorded. The pulsatility index is very high (Fig. 4-11). All these TCD patterns indirectly indicate increased intracranial pressure. Thus, TCD may not be diagnostic for brain death in patients with infratentorial lesions and in patients with brain death due to anoxic-ischemic damage. When TCD is done early, hydrocephalus or brain edema (and increased intracranial pressure) may not be present.

A consensus statement by the task force group on cerebral death of the Neurosonology Research Group of the World Federation of Neurology was published in 1998 (72) which expanded requirements.

1. Confirmation of cerebral circulatory arrest with extra- and intra-cranial Doppler sonography, bilaterally on two examinations 30 min apart.
2. Systolic spikes or oscillating flow in any cerebral artery (anterior and posterior).

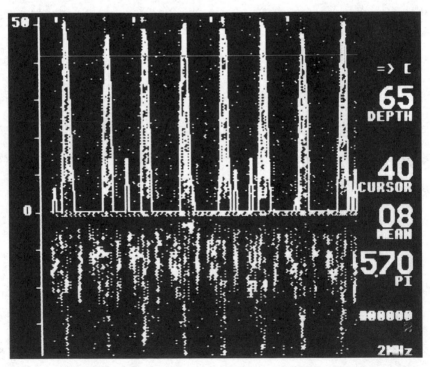

FIG. 4-11. Transcranial Doppler in brain death showing small systolic peaks and significant increase in pulsatility index.

3. Diagnosis established by intracranial examination must be confirmed by the extracranial bilateral recording of the common carotid, internal carotid, and vertebral arteries.
4. Disappearance of intracranial flow signals together with typical extracranial signs can be accepted as proof of circulatory arrest when no intracranial signal is found.
5. Exclusion of patients with ventricular drains or large craniotomy.

The major advantage of this device is its portability and the growing expertise of attending neurointensivists and neurosurgeons who may perform this study without being dependent on other technical resources.

Magnetic Resonance Imaging

Axial T_1-weighted and T_2-weighted images with spin-echo techniques, including three-dimensional time-of-flight fast imaging, have been reported (75–78). The magnetic resonance (MR) findings are transtentorial or tonsillar herniation, lack of intracranial flow void (Fig. 4-12A), poor gray-white matter differentiation, and marked contrast enhancement of the nose (MR "hot nose") and scalp (77). Proton density and T_2-weighted MR images can show dissociated intensity changes between gray and white matter.

MR angiography does not show intracranial vessels above the skull base similar to a conventional angiogram (Fig. 4-12B). There is very limited experience with this type of neuroimaging, and often studies have been interpreted retrospectively. Prospective studies in patients with evolving loss of brain function may be useful.

Single Photon Emission Computed Tomography

A single-detector rotating gamma camera is used with capabilities for monitoring and mechanical ventilation (79–84). A tracer isotope (^{99m}Tc-HMPAO) is injected intravenously 15 to 30 min before scanning. Serial pictures are taken as part of a dynamic study, followed by lateral and anterior static images with a three-dimensional image with good spatial resolution. Arrest of cerebral circulation is found in 96% of cases; in the remaining cases, perfusion may persist in the thalamus and brainstem, particularly in children. Absent uptake produces a highly characteristic "hollow skull" or "empty light bulb" phenomenon. Increased external flow may result in enhancement of the nose ("hot nose sign"; Fig. 4-13) (85,86). Absent uptake is a reflection of absent intracranial flow due to marked terminal rise in intracranial pressure, which was confirmed in 22 patients with concomitant intracranial pressure recording (86). Correlation with the cerebral angiogram is excellent.

Tracer injection may be inaccurate but can be checked with imaging of spleen uptake or assessment of the nuclear activity of the carotid arteries. Nuclear scan requires a specialist in nuclear medicine for interpretation and quality control. It is not widely available on an urgent basis.

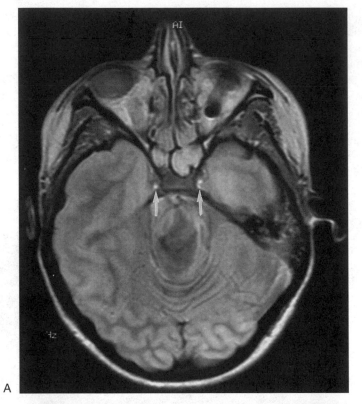

A

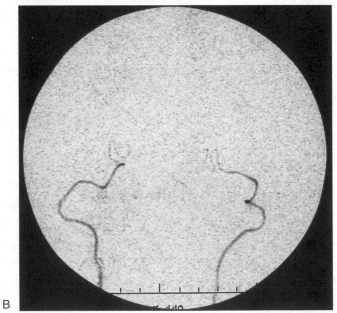

B

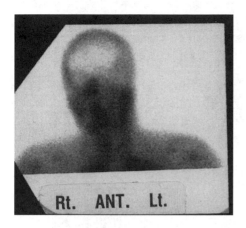

FIG. 4-13. Single photon emission computed tomography scan ("empty light bulb" or "hollow skull phenomenon"). "Hot nose sign" is a consequence of extracerebral blood flow. (By permission of the Massachusetts Medical Society.)

Evoked Potentials

Both brainstem auditory evoked potentials (BAEP) and somatosensory evoked potentials (SSEP) have been studied as potential confirmatory tests in brain death. Initial enthusiasm was fostered by examples of patients in drug-induced coma, appearing clinically to be brain dead, who had isoelectric EEGs but no change in the individual evoked components (87). Evoked potentials became a possible indicator of brainstem function in patients with major head trauma and barbiturate use.

BAEP is generated by means of bedside equipment with click intensity set at 65 dB with a 10/s stimulus repetition rate provided by earphones. It is necessary to identify wave I from the ipsilateral ear electrode to prove an intact auditory nerve, which can be destroyed as a result of cochlear trauma. Waves II and III identify the cochlear nucleus and superior olivary complex, and waves IV and V locate the upper pons; therefore, absence of waves II through V indicates profound brainstem dysfunction (88).

BAEPs are generated within the pons and do not measure tracts in the medulla oblongata. BAEPs do not correlate well with severity of brain injury. Patients with a persistent vegetative state have normal BAEPs (89), and brain-dead patients may have identifiable wave forms. Patients have been noted to have absent waves II to V after severe head injury or devastating anoxic-ischemic encephalopathy but with intact brainstem reflexes (90). Another concern is the limited number of studies with detailed clinical and laboratory correlation.

SSEPs are recorded at several sites, including second cervical vertebra and centroparietal areas with stimulation at the median nerve at the wrist at a rate of 5 Hz. Typically, approximately 2,000 responses are averaged, and the evoked potentials

---

FIG. 4-12. A: Magnetic resonance imaging in a patient fulfilling clinical criteria of brain death (after uncal herniation of a massive infarct) shows high signal in petrous portion of carotids *(arrows)*, indicating stagnation of flow. **B:** Magnetic resonance angiography showing absent intracranial flow at the skull base.

are amplified and filtered between 5 and 1,500 Hz. The recorded potentials most likely travel through the proprioceptive pathway in the spinal cord dorsal column to the medial lemniscus and to the primary somatosensory cortex. The cortical wave N20 is typically absent in brain death but is also bilaterally undetectable in approximately 15% to 20% of patients who are comatose but not brain dead. Recent studies suggest that disappearance of the P14 wave (bulbomedullary junction or cuneate nucleus) may be helpful. Distinction from artifacts is difficult, but nasopharyngeal electrode recording of P14 may enhance its detection, only to disappear when brain death occurs. Experience is limited.

Sonoo and co-workers (91) directed attention to the value of the N18 potential possibly generated in the cuneate nucleus, but it was also absent in 3 of 20 comatose patients who were not brain dead. The relatively poor predictive value casts doubt on the use of the BAEP or SSEP as a standard confirmatory test for brain death (92–102).

Spiral Computed Tomography Scan

Spiral CT scan has the advantage of allowing evaluation of the intracranial circulation through intravenous injection of contrast (103–105). Circulatory arrest was present in a preliminary study of 14 patients with no flow in the basilar artery, posterior cerebral arteries, pericallosal arteries, and terminal cortical arteries but weak visualization in the M1 segment of the middle cerebral artery and A1 segment of the anterior cerebral artery. There is no other recent published experience.

CONCLUSION

Clinical neurologic examination in brain death prevails over any technologic investigation. Its reliability has been tested over the years, errors in interpretation are exceptional, and observer agreement is excellent. Change in neurologic examination has not occurred in adults when conducted properly, but observation over time is advised. The apnea test can be performed in a very simplified manner without major complications if oxygenation is guaranteed. The complete determination of this state, however, may best fit in a neurologic or neurosurgical practice.

REFERENCES

1. The Quality Standards Subcommittee of the American Academy of Neurology. Practice parameters for determining brain death in adults (summary statement). *Neurology* 1995;45:1012–1014.
2. Wijdicks EFM. Determining brain death in adults. *Neurology* 1995;45:1003–1011.
3. Wijdicks EFM. Temporomandibular joint compression in coma. *Neurology* 1996;46:1774.
4. Santamaria J, Orteu N, Iranzo A, et al. Eye opening in brain death [Letter]. *J Neurol* 1999; 246:720–722.
5. Friedman AJ. Sympathetic response and brain death [Letter]. *Arch Neurol* 1984;41:15.
6. Sims JK, Bickford RG. Non-mydriatic pupils occurring in human brain death. *Bull LA Neurol Soc* 1973;38:24–32.
7. Greenan J, Prasad J. Comparison of the ocular effects of atropine or glycopyrrolate with two I.V. induction agents. *Br J Anaesth* 1985;57:180–183.

8. Goetting MG, Contreras E. Systemic atropine administration during cardiac arrest does not cause fixed and dilated pupils. *Ann Emerg Med* 1991;20:55–57.
9. Gray AT, Krejci ST, Larson MD. Neuromuscular blocking drugs do not alter the pupillary light reflex of anesthetized humans. *Arch Neurol* 1997;54:579–584.
10. Schmidt JE, Tamburro RF, Hoffman GM. Dilated nonreactive pupils secondary to neuromuscular blockade. *Anesthesiology* 2000;92:1476–1480.
11. Snavely SR, Hodges GR. The neurotoxicity of antibacterial agents. *Ann Intern Med* 1984; 101:92–104.
12. Draper WB, Whitehead RW. Diffusion respiration in dog anesthetized by pentothal sodium. *Anesthesiology* 1944;5:262–273.
13. al Jumah M, McLean DR, al Rajeh S, et al. Bulk diffusion apnea test in the diagnosis of brain death. *Crit Care Med* 1992;20:1564–1567.
14. Feery JJ, Waller GA, Solliday N. The use of apneic-diffusion respiration in the diagnosis of brain death. *Respir Care* 1985;30:328–333.
15. Ferris EB, Engel GL, Stevens CD, et al. Voluntary breathholding; the relation of the maximum time of breathholding to the oxygen and carbon dioxide tensions of arterial blood, with a note on its clinical and physiological significance. *J Clin Invest* 1946;25:734–743.
16. Bruce EN, Cherniack NS. Central chemoreceptors. *J Appl Physiol* 1987;62:389–402.
17. Joels N, Samueloff M. The activity of the medullary centres in diffusion respiration. *J Physiol* 1956; 133:360–372.
18. Lang CJ. Apnea testing by artificial CO_2 augmentation. *Neurology* 1995;45:966–969.
19. Rohling R, Wagner W, Mühlberg J, et al. Apnea test: pitfalls and correct handling. *Transplant Proc* 1986;18:388–390.
20. Jeret JS, Benjamin JL. Risk of hypotension during apnea testing. *Arch Neurol* 1994;51:595–599.
21. Coimbra CG. Implications of ischemic penumbra for the diagnosis of brain death. *Braz J Med Biol Res* 1999;32:1479–1487.
22. Goudreau JL, Wijdicks EFM, Emery SF. Complications during apnea testing in the determination of brain death: predisposing factors. *Neurology* 2000;55:1045–1048.
23. Eger EI, Severinghaus JW. The rate of rise of $Paco_2$ in the apneic anesthetized patient. *Anesthesiology* 1961;22:419–425.
24. Engel GL, Ferris EB, Webb JP, et al. Voluntary breathholding; the relation of the maximum time of breathholding to the oxygen tension of the inspired air. *J Clin Invest* 1946;25:729–733.
25. Marks SJ, Zisfein J. Apneic oxygenation in apnea tests for brain death. A controlled trial. *Arch Neurol* 1990;47:1066–1068.
26. Prechter GC, Nelson SB, Hubmayr RD. The ventilatory recruitment threshold for carbon dioxide. *Am Rev Respir Dis* 1990;141:758–764.
27. Hanks EC, Ngai SH, Fink BR. The respiratory threshold for carbon dioxide in anesthetized man. Determination of carbon dioxide threshold during halothane anesthesia. *Anesthesiology* 1961; 22:393–397.
28. Ropper AH, Kennedy SK, Russel L. Apnea testing in the diagnosis of brain death: clinical and physiological observations. *J Neurosurg* 1981;55:942–946.
29. Wijdicks EFM. In search of a safe apnea test in brain death: Is the procedure really more dangerous than we think? [Letter]. *Arch Neurol* 1995;52:338–339.
30. Benzel EC, Mashburn JP, Conrad S, et al. Apnea testing for the determination of brain death: a modified protocol [Technical note]. *J Neurosurg* 1992;76:1029–1031.
31. Orliaguet GA, Catoire P, Liu N, et al. Transesophageal echocardiographic assessment of left ventricular function during apnea testing for brain death. *Transplantation* 1994;58:655–658.
32. Goulon M, Nouailhat F, Babinet P. Irreversible coma [French]. *Ann Med Interne (Paris)* 1971; 122:479–486.
33. Hanna JP, Frank JI. Automatic stepping in the pontomedullary stage of central herniation. *Neurology* 1995;45:985–986.
34. Bueri JA, Saposnik G, Maurino J, et al. Lazarus' sign in brain death. *Mov Disord* 2000;15:583–586.
35. Christie JM, O'Lenic TD, Cane RD. Head turning in brain death. *J Clin Anesth* 1996;8:141–143.
36. Saposnik G, Bueri JA, Maurino J, et al. Spontaneous and reflex movements in brain death. *Neurology* 2000;54:221–223.
37. Ropper AH. Unusual spontaneous movements in brain-dead patients. *Neurology* 1984; 34:1089–1092.
38. Martí-Fàbregas J, López-Navidad A, Caballero F, et al. Decerebrate-like posturing with mechanical ventilation in brain death. *Neurology* 2000;54:224–227.

39. McNair NL, Meador KJ. The undulating toe flexion sign in brain death. *Mov Disord* 1992; 7:345–347.
40. Walker AE, Feeney DM, Hovda DA. The electroencephalographic characteristics of the rhomben-cephalectomized cat. *Electroencephalogr Clin Neurophysiol* 1984;57:156–165.
41. Cantu RC. Brain death as determined by cerebral arteriography [Letter]. *Lancet* 1973;1:1391–1392.
42. Wijdicks EFM. What anesthesiologists should know about what neurologists should know about declaring brain death [Letter]. *Anesthesiology* 2000;92:1203–1204.
43. Van Norman GA. A matter of life and death: what every anesthesiologist should know about the medical, legal, and ethical aspects of declaring brain death. *Anesthesiology* 1999;91:275–287.
44. Koberda JL, Clark WM, Lutsep H, et al. Successful clinical recovery and reversal of mid-basilar occlusion in clinically brain dead patient with intra-arterial urokinase [Abstract]. *Neurology* 1997; 48:A154.
45. López-Navidad A, Caballero F, Domingo P, et al. Early diagnosis of brain death in patients treated with central nervous system depressant drugs. *Transplantation* 2000;70:131–135.
46. Bergquist E, Bergstrom K. Angiography in cerebral death. *Acta Radiol* 1972;12:283–288.
47. Korein J, Braunstein P, George A, et al. Brain death: I. Angiographic correlation with the radioisotopic bolus technique for evaluation of critical deficit of cerebral blood flow. *Ann Neurol* 1977; 2:195–205.
48. Korein J, Braunstein P, Kricheff I, et al. Radioisotopic bolus technique as a test to detect circulatory deficit associated with cerebral death. 142 studies on 80 patients demonstrating the bedside use of an innocuous IV procedure as an adjunct in the diagnosis of cerebral death. *Circulation* 1975; 51:924–939.
49. Kricheff II, Pinto RS, George AE, et al. Angiographic findings in brain death. *Ann NY Acad Sci* 1978; 315:168–183.
50. Greitz T, Gordon E, Kolmodin G, et al. Aortocranial and carotid angiography in determination of brain death. *Neuroradiology* 1973;5:13–19.
51. Hazratji SM, Singh BM, Strobos RJ. Angiography in brain death. *NYS J Med* 1981;81:82–83.
52. Bradac GB, Simon RS. Angiography in brain death. *Neuroradiology* 1974;7:25–28.
53. Jefferson NR, Ameratunga B, Rajapakse S. Angiographic evidence of brain death. *Australas Radiol* 1975;19:289–296.
54. Langfitt TW, Kassell NF. Non-filling of cerebral vessels during angiography: correlation with intracranial pressure. *Acta Neurochir* 1966;14:96–104.
55. Deliyannakis E, Ioannou F, Davaroukas A. Brain stem death with persistence of bioelectric activity of the cerebral hemispheres. *Clin Electroencephalogr* 1975;6:75–79.
56. Hughes JR. Limitations of the EEG in coma and brain death. *Ann NY Acad Sci* 1978;315:121–136.
57. Jorgensen EO. Technical contribution. Requirements for recording the EEG at high sensitivity in suspected brain death. *Electrocephalogr Clin Neurophysiol* 1974;36:65–69.
58. Bennett DR. The EEG in determination of brain death. *Ann NY Acad Sci* 1978;315:110–120.
59. Grigg MM, Kelly MA, Celesia GG, et al. Electroencephalographic activity after brain death. *Arch Neurol* 1987;44:948–954.
60. American Electroencephalographic Society. Guideline three: minimum technical standards for EEG recording in suspected cerebral death. *J Clin Neurophysiol* 1994;11:10–13.
61. Silverman D, Saunders MG, Schwab RS, et al. Cerebral death and the electroencephalogram. Report of the ad hoc committee of the American Electroencephalographic Society on EEG Criteria for Determination of Cerebral Death. *JAMA* 1969;209:1505–1510.
62. Buchner H, Schuchardt V. Reliability of electroencephalogram in the diagnosis of brain death. *Eur Neurol* 1990;30:138–141.
63. Hassler W, Steinmetz H, Gawlowski J. Transcranial Doppler ultrasonography in raised intracranial pressure and in intracranial circulatory arrest. *J Neurosurg* 1988;68:745–751.
64. Klingelhofer J, Conrad B, Benecke R, et al. Evaluation of intracranial pressure from transcranial Doppler studies in cerebral disease. *J Neurol* 1988;235:159–162.
65. Report of the American Academy of Neurology, Therapeutics and Technology Assessment Subcommittee. Assessment: transcranial Doppler. *Neurology* 1990;40:680–681.
66. Feri M, Ralli L, Felici M, et al. Transcranial Doppler and brain death diagnosis. *Crit Care Med* 1994; 22:1120–1126.
67. Powers AD, Graeber MC, Smith RR. Transcranial Doppler ultrasonography in the determination of brain death. *Neurosurgery* 1989;24:884–889.
68. Van Velthoven V, Calliauw L. Diagnosis of brain death. Transcranial Doppler sonography as an additional method. *Acta Neurochir* 1988;95:57–60.

69. Hadani M, Bruk B, Ram Z, et al. Application of transcranial Doppler ultrasonography for the diagnosis of brain death. *Intensive Care Med* 1999;25:822–828.
70. Saunders FW, Cledgett P. Intracranial blood velocity in head injury. A transcranial ultrasound Doppler study. *Surg Neurol* 1988;29:401–409.
71. Ducrocq X, Braun M, Debouveric M, et al. Brain death and transcranial Doppler: experience in 130 cases of brain dead patients. *J Neurol Sci* 1998;160:41–46.
72. Ducrocq X, Hassler W, Moritake K, et al. Consensus opinion on diagnosis of cerebral circulatory arrest using Doppler-sonography: Task Force Group on Cerebral Death of the Neurosonology Research Group of the World Federation of Neurology. *J Neurol Sci* 1998;159:145–150.
73. Petty GW, Mohr JP, Pedley TA, et al. The role of transcranial Doppler in confirming brain death: sensitivity, specificity, and suggestions for performance and interpretation. *Neurology* 1990; 40:300–303.
74. Ropper AH, Kehne SM, Wechsler L. Transcranial Doppler in brain death. *Neurology* 1987; 37:1733–1735.
75. Ishii K, Onuma T, Kinoshita T, et al. Brain death: MR and MR angiography. *AJNR Am J Neuroradiol* 1996;17:731–735.
76. Matsumura A, Mequero K, Tsurushima H, et al. Magnetic resonance imaging of brain death. *Neurol Med Clin Chir* 1996;36:166–171.
77. Orrison WW Jr, Champlin AM, Kesterson OL, et al. MR "hot nose sign" and "intravascular enhancement sign" in brain death. *AJNR Am J Neuroradiol* 1994;15:913–916.
78. Lee DH, Nathanson JA, Fox AJ, et al. Magnetic resonance imaging of brain death. *Can Assoc Radiol J* 1995;46:174–178.
79. Roine RO, Launes J, Lindroth L, et al. ^{99m}Tc-hexamethylpropyleneamine oxime scans to confirm brain death [Letter]. *Lancet* 1986;2:1223–1224.
80. Yatim A, Mercatello A, Caronel B, et al. ^{99m}Tc-HMPAO cerebral scintigraphy in the diagnosis of brain death. *Transplant Proc* 1991;23:2491.
81. George MS. Establishing brain death: the potential role of nuclear medicine in the search for a reliable confirmatory test [Editorial]. *Eur J Nucl Med* 1991;18:75–77.
82. Laurin NR, Driedger AA, Hurwitz GA, et al. Cerebral perfusion imaging with technetium-99m HM-PAO in brain death and severe central nervous system injury. *J Nucl Med* 1989;30: 1627–1635.
83. Bonetti MG, Ciritella P, Valle G, et al. ^{99m}Tc HM-PAO brain perfusion SPECT in brain death. *Neuroradiology* 1995;37:365–369.
84. Facco E, Zucchetta P, Munari M, et al. ^{99m}Tc-HMPAO SPECT in the diagnosis of brain death. *Intensive Care Med* 1998;24:911–917.
85. Mishkin FS, Dyken ML. Increased early radionuclide activity in the nasopharyngeal area in patients with internal carotid artery obstruction: "hot nose." *Radiology* 1970;96:77–80.
86. Kurtek RW, Lai KK, Tauxe WN, et al. Tc-99m hexamethylpropylene amine oxime scintigraphy in the diagnosis of brain death and its implications for the harvesting of organs used for transplantation. *Clin Nucl Med* 2000;25:7–10.
87. Sharbrough FW. Unique contributions of short-latency auditory and somatosensory evoked potentials to neurologic diagnosis. *Prog Clin Neurophysiol* 1980;7:231–263.
88. Chiappa KH, ed. *Evoked potentials in clinical medicine,* 3rd ed. Philadelphia: Lippincott–Raven Publishers, 1997.
89. Hansotia PL. Persistent vegetative state. Review and report of electrodiagnostic studies in eight cases. *Arch Neurol* 1985;42:1048–1052.
90. Brunko E, Delecluse F, Herbaut AG, et al. Unusual pattern of somatosensory and brain-stem auditory evoked potentials after cardiorespiratory arrest. *Electroencephalogr Clin Neurophysiol* 1985; 62:338–342.
91. Sonoo M, Tsai-Shozawa Y, Aoki M, et al. N18 in median somatosensory evoked potentials: a new indicator of medullary function useful for the diagnosis of brain death. *J Neurol Neurosurg Psychiatry* 1999;67:374–378.
92. Roncucci P, Lepori P, Mok MS, et al. Nasopharyngeal electrode recording of somatosensory evoked potentials as an indicator in brain death. *Anaesth Intensive Care* 1999;27:20–25.
93. Anziska BJ, Cracco RQ. Short latency somatosensory evoked potentials in brain dead patients. *Arch Neurol* 1980;37:222–225.
94. Firsching R. The brain-stem and 40 Hz middle latency auditory evoked potentials in brain death. *Acta Neurochir* 1989;101:52–55.

95. Garcia-Larrea L, Bertrand O, Artru F, et al. Brain-stem monitoring. II. Preterminal BAEP changes observed until brain death in deeply comatose patients. *Electroencephalogr Clin Neurophysiol* 1987; 68:446–457.

96. Stohr M, Riffel B, Trost E, et al. Short-latency somatosensory evoked potentials in brain death. *J Neurol* 1987;234:211–214.

97. Starr A. Auditory brain-stem responses in brain death. *Brain* 1976;99:543–554.

98. Wagner W. SEP testing in deeply comatose and brain dead patients: the role of nasopharyngeal, scalp and earlobe derivations in recording the P14 potential. *Electroencephalogr Clin Neurophysiol* 1991; 80:352–363.

99. Goldie WD, Chiappa KH, Young RR, et al. Brainstem auditory and short-latency somatosensory evoked responses in brain death. *Neurology* 1981;31:248–256.

100. Chancellor AM, Frith RW, Shaw NA. Somatosensory evoked potentials following severe head injury: loss of the thalamic potential with brain death. *J Neurol Sci* 1988;87:255–263.

101. Belsh JM, Chokroverty S. Short-latency somatosensory evoked potentials in brain-dead patients. *Electroencephalogr Clin Neurophysiol* 1987;68:75–78.

102. Machado C, Valdés P, García-Tigera J, et al. Brain-stem auditory evoked potentials and brain death. *Electroencephalogr Clin Neurophysiol* 1991;80:392–398.

103. Arnold H, Kunhe D, Rohr W, et al. Contrast bolus technique with rapid CT scanning. A reliable diagnostic tool for the determination of brain death. *Neuroradiology* 1981;22:129–132.

104. Rangel RA. Computerized axial tomography in brain death. *Stroke* 1978;9:597–598.

105. Dupas B, Gayet-Delacroix M, Villers D, et al. Diagnosis of brain death using two-phase spiral CT. *AJNR Am J Neuroradiol* 1998;19:641–647.

5

Clinical Diagnosis and Confirmatory Testing of Brain Death in Children

Stephen Ashwal

Division of Pediatric Neurology, Loma Linda University School of Medicine, Loma Linda, California

The diagnosis of brain death in pediatric patients is based on the same principles as in adults. But the neurologic examination is more difficult to perform and interpret because of the smaller size of the patient, immaturity of certain development reflexes being tested, and pathophysiologic differences due to the presence of open sutures and fontanels in the neonate and infant.

Brain death most commonly occurs in children less than 1 year of age and is uncommon in adolescents. Brain death in children is most frequently due to traumatic brain injury from abuse (e.g., shaken baby syndrome) and less often from motor vehicle accidents. Asphyxia is a comparatively common circumstance surrounding brain death in children and occurs after near drowning, from strangulation or suffocation, or from sudden infant death syndrome (SIDS). Brain death secondary to inflammatory diseases such as fulminant encephalitis and meningitis may be complicated by massive cerebral edema with the onset of brain herniation within 1 day of hospitalization. Much less common causes of brain death are metabolic diseases, perioperative central nervous system insults, and acute obstructive hydrocephalus.

Studies from pediatric intensive care units in the past decade have reported that older infants and children with brain death are a very small number of admissions (Table 5-1). There is a marked variation between institutions and this likely reflects differences in ascertainment. Two Canadian studies have reported mortality data from neonatal and pediatric intensive care units. The mortality rate in the pediatric intensive care unit (PICU) approximated 9%, with 22% of these children declared brain dead (1). Mortality rate in the neonatal intensive care unit (NICU) was almost 6% with none of the infants declared brain dead (1). More recently, Parker and co-investigators reported the percentage of brain deaths to overall deaths to be 31% in children over 1 month of age and 6% in neonates (2). Our data from Loma Linda University Children's Hospital over the past several years found the percentage of brain deaths to overall deaths to be 28% and 2%, respectively, in our pediatric and neonatal units. In some PICUs, the percent of patients diagnosed as brain dead compared to all deaths is even higher (i.e., up to 38%) (3,4).

TABLE 5-1. *Incidence of brain death in older children and neonates*

	Patients >1 mo				Neonates (<30 d of age)			
Study	No. of patients	Mortality rate (%)	Percentage of patients brain dead compared to total	Percentage of patients brain dead compared to death	No. of patients	Mortality rate (%)	Percentage of neonates brain dead compared to total	Percentage of neonates brain dead compared to death
Rowland et al., 1983 (7)	2,307	NA	0.65	NA	NA	NA	NA	NA
Vernon et al., 1993	6,000	5.0	1.2	23.3	NA	NA	NA	NA
Ryan et al., 1993 (1)	839	8.7	1.2	22	1,333	5.6	0	0
Staworn et al., 1994	14,188	8.5	0.9	11	NA	NA	NA	NA
Parker et al., 1995 (2)	2,605	6.5	2.0	31.4	1,455	7.6	0.48	6.3
Loma Linda, 2000*	5,093	5.0	1.3	28.1	2,977	6.2	0.02	2.1

Time period refers to the duration of the study. For several studies, separation of the data by neonates versus older pediatric patients was not possible. In the study by Parker et al. (2), there were seven neonates less than 30 days old, six of whom were less than 7 days old (personal correspondence).
* Ashwal S (personal experience, unpublished data).

Declaration and confirmation of brain death in the majority of pediatric patients presenting in coma after a serious central nervous system injury are usually completed within the first 2 days of hospitalization (5,6). If not referred for organ donation, these children are subsequently removed from life support systems once the diagnosis of brain death is confirmed (5,6). Rarely, brain-dead pediatric patients have been maintained with ventilator support because cardiac arrest occurred with an average of about 17 days. Longer survival has been claimed by Shewmon after an exhaustive review of the literature and personally examined cases (for detailed discussion, see Chapter 9).

There have been no reports of children recovering neurologic function who met adult brain death criteria on neurologic examination (7–9). In 1987, guidelines for the determination of brain death in children in the United States were proposed by a Task Force (10) that represented several of the major professional medical and legal societies (Table 5-2). These guidelines emphasized the importance of the history and clinical examination in determining the etiology of coma in order to eliminate reversible conditions. In addition, age-related observation periods and the need for specific neurodiagnostic tests were recommended for children below the age of 1 year. In children older than 1 year, it was recommended that the diagnosis of brain death could be made solely on a clinical basis and laboratory studies were optional. Since publication in 1987, these explicit guidelines have been generally accepted (11,12). At the time these guidelines were developed, criteria for term infants less than 7 days of age and preterm infants were excluded because of the lack of sufficient data. More

TABLE 5-2. *Guidelines for brain death determination in children*

A. History: determine the cause of coma to eliminate reversible conditions
B. Physical examination criteria:
  1. Coma and apnea
  2. Absence of brainstem function
    (a) Midposition or fully dilated pupils
    (b) Absence of spontaneous oculocephalic (doll's eye) and caloric-induced eye movements
    (c) Absence of movement of bulbar musculature, corneal, gag, cough, sucking, and rooting reflexes
    (d) Absence of respiratory effort with standardized testing for apnea
  3. Patient must not be hypothermic or hypotensive
  4. Flaccid tone and absence of spontaneous or induced movements, excluding activity mediated at spinal cord level
  5. Examination should remain consistent for brain death throughout the predetermined period of observation
C. Observation period according to age:
  1. 7 days to 2 months: Two examinations and EEGs 48 h apart
  2. 2 months to 1 year: Two examinations and EEGs 24 h apart or one examination and an initial EEG showing ECS combined with a radionuclide angiogram showing no CBF, or both
  3. More than 1 year: Two examinations 12–24 h apart; EEG and isotope angiography are optional

The Ad Hoc Task Force consisted of representatives from the Academy of Pediatrics, American Academy of Neurology, Child Neurology Society, American Neurological Association, American Bar Association, and the NINCDS.
From Guidelines for the determination of brain death in children. *Pediatrics* 1987;80:298–300, with permission.

recent studies have found that criteria used in infants under age 2 months can also be applied to preterm and term infants (13–15) (Fig. 5-1).

Guideline dissemination remains problematic; that is, many physicians who care for children are not sufficiently aware of the specific diagnostic criteria recommended by the Task Force. For example, in one recent survey using fictional cases, only 36% of pediatric residents and 39% of pediatric attending physicians correctly defined brain death and only 58% of residents or attending physicians recognized that brain death in certain age brackets could be determined without confirmatory testing (16). Likewise, a survey of pediatric intensivists reported a wide variability in their use of confirmatory laboratory tests (17). Forty-one percent of respondents to this survey never considered use of the electroencephalogram (EEG) and 33% never considered use of cerebral blood flow (CBF) determinations for confirmation of brain death. Also, although 69% of respondents stated that more than one physician was required to make the diagnosis of brain death, 19% stated that one physician was sufficient and in only 71% of situations was either a neurologist or a neurosurgeon consistently involved.

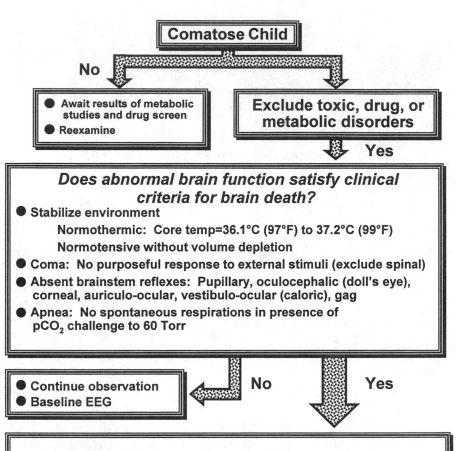

FIG. 5-1. Diagnostic paradigm for the determination of brain death in neonates, infants and children based on the 1987 Pediatric Brain Death Guidelines (Table 5-2) (10) modified to include newborn infants.

CLINICAL EXAMINATION

By definition, all children who are declared brain dead are comatose, lack brainstem reflexes, and are apneic. These criteria may not be present on admission in all children who ultimately are declared brain dead (18), and often are fulfilled after serial examinations. As in adults, reversible conditions associated with hypothermia, altered metabolic states, toxin exposure, severe electrolyte abnormalities, or sedative medication should be excluded. It should be emphasized that hypothermia occurs in about 50% of children who are comatose after catastrophic brain injury, and there is a common need to rewarm the child before neurologic examination and neurodiagnostic tests. It may also prolong the elimination of drugs, if any have been administered soon before assessment.

Coma

Assessment of the lack of consciousness may be difficult in infants and children. Although there is no absolute way to be completely certain that a neonate or young infant has lost all conscious awareness and is "unreceptive and unresponsive" as stated in the original Task Force criteria, testing by tactile, visual, and auditory stimulation is comparable to the older infant. In most instances and irrespective of the age of the child, the bedside clinical examination can satisfactorily accomplish this goal. The absence of any form of repetitive, sustained purposeful activity should be documented (19). If there is uncertainty that the child is unresponsive, confirmatory neurodiagnostic studies should be performed.

Loss of Brainstem Function

In preterm and term neonates one must take into account that several of the brainstem reflexes are not fully developed (20–22) (Table 5-3). For example, the pupil-

TABLE 5-3. *Development of reflexes in preterm infants*

Developmental reflex	Gestational age (weeks) when reflex is elicitable
Suck, root, gag	32–34
Auditory response	30–32
Pupillary response to light	30–32
Oculocephalic response	28–32
Corneal response	28–32
Moro response	28–32
Grasp response	34–36
Breathing response to P_{CO_2} stimulus	33

From Fanaroff A, Martin RJ, Miller MJ. The respiratory system. In: Fanaroff A, Martin RJ, eds. *Neonatal-perinatal medicine: diseases of the fetus and newborn.* St. Louis: CV Mosby, 1987:617; Hack M. The sensorimotor development of the preterm infant. In: Fanaroff A, Martin RJ, eds. *Neonatal-perinatal medicine: diseases of the fetus and newborn.* St. Louis: CV Mosby, 1987:473; and Swaiman KF. Neurological examination of the preterm infant. In: Swaiman KF, ed. *Pediatric neurology: principles and practice.* St. Louis: Mosby, 1994:61, with permission.

lary light reflex is absent before 30 weeks gestation and the oculocephalic reflex may not be elicitable prior to 32 weeks. Term and preterm infants are difficult to examine because their small size makes it technically difficult to adequately assess cranial nerve function. The smaller amount of pigmentation and the smaller size of the newborn's pupils can make visualization of changes in the size of the pupil and interpretation of the loss of pupillary reactivity troublesome. In addition, assessment of pupillary reactivity can be compromised at the bedside from difficult access to the infant in an incubator, corneal injury, retinal hemorrhages and other anatomical factors such as swelling with partial fusion of the eyelids. Examination of ocular motility is difficult in the small intubated child and frequently the examiner will need assistance when performing caloric stimulation with ice water. It is more difficult to perform the caloric response in neonates due to small external ear canals; therefore, both the oculocephalic (doll's eye) and the oculovestibular (caloric) reflex should be tested. There are no substantial differences in performing this testing in newborns compared to older children (see Chapter 4).

The corneal reflex in neonates and infants is potentially the least reliable. Contact irritation, dehydration and maceration of the cornea, use of lubricant drops, and use of eye patches for treatment of hyperbilirubinemia frequently negatively affect tactile surface sensory receptors of the cornea. A noxious stimulus with a soaked Q-tip may be needed.

Assessment of lower cranial nerve function is also limited. There may be a substantial amount of adhesive tape around the face and cheek to secure the endotracheal tube and this impedes the clinician's ability to perform this part of the neurologic assessment, similar to adults. When infants are intubated (either by the oral or nasogastric route), testing their gag and cough reflex is best accomplished with stimulation of the trachea after inserting of a suction catheter through the endotracheal tube.

Apnea

The normal physiologic threshold for apnea (minimum carbon dioxide tension at which respiratory centers are maximally stimulated) can be altered by certain disease states, but the threshold ($PaCO_2 \geq 60$ mm Hg) for children has been assumed to be the same as that for adults (2,23,24).

Several studies have examined apnea testing in children with varying techniques. In one study of 10 brain-dead children (10 months to 15 years of age), the $PaCO_2$ was increased from 34.4 mm Hg to 59.5 mm Hg over 5 min while supplying 100% tracheal oxygen, which maintained the arterial PO_2 greater than 200 mm Hg during the test period (24). None of the children had any evidence of respiratory effort. A second study involved 16 apnea tests in nine children ages 4 months to 13 years, four of whom had detectable phenobarbital levels between 10 and 25 mg/dL (23). These patients were preoxygenated (100% O_2) for 10 min and moderately hyperventilated (mean $PaCO_2$ 28 mm Hg). Oxygen was then delivered at 6 L/min through a catheter into the length of the endotracheal tube with the ventilator turned off during the 15-min study period. The $PaCO_2$ increased 4.4, 3.4, and 2.6 mm Hg per minute at 5, 10, and 15 min, respectively.

Arterial $Paco_2$ at the end of 15 min ranged from 40 to 116 mm Hg, and by 15 min, 14 of 16 patients had $Paco_2$ levels greater than 60 mm Hg. Two patients had $Paco_2$ levels of 110 and 116 mm Hg (pH of 6.92 and 6.98, respectively). Arterial Po_2 remained above 100 mm Hg in all patients and in 12 of 16 patients was above 200 mm Hg. Mild alterations of heart rate or blood pressure or both were also observed in six patients but were reversible. A third study in 11 children found that if apnea testing was done when the initial $Paco_2$ level was between 40 and 50 mm Hg, the rate of $Paco_2$ increase was linear at 5.1 to 6.7 mm Hg per minute (25). Parker and colleagues reviewed data on apnea testing in 60 brain-dead children (2). Nine patients who also had EEGs showed electroencephalographic silence and 26 of 30 patients who had CBF studies had no flow. These children were preoxygenated for 10 min followed by continuous oxygen delivery (6 L/min). The median $Paco_2$ at the end of testing was 74 mm Hg (range, 55 to 112). None of these patients showed any recovery of respiratory drive.

Recent reports concerning apnea testing in children have raised questions about (a) the effects of brainstem compressive lesions; (b) potential recovery of brainstem respiratory drive; and (c) the $Paco_2$ threshold in children. Ammar and colleagues in 1993 reported five children, ages 9 months to 7 years. In these patients, severe brainstem dysfunction included loss of pupillary reflexes and apnea and was due to surgically resectable brainstem lesions. Spontaneous respirations and substantial neurologic function returned after surgery (26). This report suggested that treatment of compressive brainstem lesions might reverse severe neurologic deficits that mimic brain death. However, none of these children were brain dead prior to surgery. Another report is that of a 3-month-old infant who met the 1987 Task Force criteria for pediatric brain death but who on day 43 of hospitalization developed two to three irregular breaths per minute with a normal tidal volume (27). This infant died 71 days after presentation. At issue is whether this should be considered a return of respiratory function and, if true, whether return of irregular breathing in a single exceptional case in the absence of other brainstem function is an "improvement". An editorial commentary on this study did not accept this as an example of failure of current brain death criteria, and we agree (28).

The $Paco_2$ threshold for maximal stimulation of the medullary centers was examined in a case report involving a 4-year-old child with a posterior fossa pilocytic astrocytoma who suffered a cardiac arrest (29). This child met clinical criteria for brain death but had minimal respiratory effort after 9 min and 23 s into the apnea test. Arterial $Paco_2$ measured 91 mm Hg and the exhaled tidal volumes of 5 to 7 mL/kg were considered true spontaneous respiratory efforts. He showed "minimal brain stem recovery" and was discharged to a chronic care facility with a gastrostomy and tracheostomy with mechanical ventilation but without return of consciousness. This child's spontaneous breathing was insufficient to maintain life and assisted ventilation was necessary. It was speculated that this child's higher $Paco_2$ threshold was due to hypoxic-ischemic injury. This example raises questions whether the current standard of a $Paco_2$ of 60 mm Hg is correct in children. However, no prospective studies have appeared with prolonged apneic oxygenation (6) and, as alluded to earlier, prior examples have not shown appearance of respiratory drive at very high levels of $Paco_2$

(23). These isolated incidences are of interest but do not seriously challenge the conventional thinking that apnea testing, aiming at acute substantial increase in $Paco_2$, is the best method in children.

The technique of apnea testing is identical as in adults using apneic oxygenation after disconnecting from the ventilator. Therefore, normalization of the $Paco_2$, core temperature, and preoxygenation for 5 min before beginning the apnea challenge is recommended. Careful monitoring of the heart rate and blood pressure during the procedure while watching the chest cage for movements is needed. Most studies recommend that $Paco_2$ levels be determined at 5-min intervals and continue for 15 min if the $Paco_2$ has not reached 60 mm Hg and if the Po_2 has not fallen below 50 mm Hg. However, calculation of time to target level assuming a $Paco_2$ rise of 3 mm Hg per minute may reduce blood gas sampling and is preferred. The technique of apnea testing is illustrated in Chapter 4. Prolonged bradycardia or development of hypotension during testing is mostly due to profound acidosis or hypoxemia; and at this juncture, the infant should be placed back on the ventilator.

CONFIRMATORY TESTS

EEG documentation of electrocerebral silence (ECS) and measurement of the absence of CBF remain the most widely available and useful methods to confirm the clinical diagnosis of brain death. However, over the past decade, there has been a trend in children to rely more upon repeated clinical examinations than to use confirmatory testing.

Electroencephalography

Guidelines for recordings in brain death have been developed by the American Electroencephalographic Society in 1994 (30) and are summarized in Chapter 4. However, certain unique aspects of electroencephalography (EEG) recording must be considered in confirming the diagnosis of brain death in neonates and infants (8,14,31–35). This includes: shorter interelectrode distances reducing detection of very-low-voltage activity; external artifacts in NICUs and PICUs brought on due to high gain settings; rapid cardiac and respiratory rates of infants and children compared to adults; shorter distances between the heart and the brain making the electrocardiogram contribution disproportionately large in children; reduced amplitude of cortical potentials in preterm and term neonates; and the presence of congenital cerebral nervous system malformations (e.g., hydranencephaly) that can be associated with ECS (36).

It is well recognized that a certain number of brain-dead infants and children will have persistent EEG activity (37–39). Most of these EEG patterns depict low-voltage theta or beta activity or intermittent spindle activity. Although electrocortical activity is generated in dying cortical cells, its persistence in otherwise functionally dead brains may continue for days. Moreover, data from several studies have found that the initial EEG in brain-dead children is isoelectric in as low as 48% of patients (Table 5-4). However, in the majority of children who initially have EEG activity, follow-up studies show ECS.

Conversely, when the initial EEG in children demonstrates ECS, a repeat EEG typically will remain isoelectric (8,39). However, there have been reported cases of recovery of EEG activity. In some reports, the EEG findings were either inconclusive or the patients had some retained brainstem function and thus did not meet clinical criteria for brain death. It remains unclear in some cases whether the EEGs were not artifactual (14). Since Green and Lauber's report almost 30 years ago of two infants who had return of some EEG activity after initial ECS, there have been five additional reports in infants in whom EEG activity returned (14,31,37,40). None of these infants recovered any neurologic function. The ratio of these five infants (i.e., in whom the initial EEG was isoelectric but the second EEG showed activity) to the number of neonatal and pediatric patients diagnosed as brain dead in published reports since 1972 is approximately 5/22,500 or 0.02% (15). Therefore, concerns about the return of EEG activity have been overemphasized, and the impact of these observations on brain death recommendations is very uncertain and likely inconsequential. None of these five infants recovered and not even to a vegetative or minimally conscious state.

It should be emphasized that electroencephalographic silence may occur soon after a child has had a cardiac arrest (41). In infants in whom the initial EEG, 8 to 10 h after cardiac arrest, showed an isoelectric recording, a repeat study 12 to 24 h later may show diffuse low-voltage activity. Most of these infants, none fulfilling clinical criteria of brain death, die from associated complications of the acute catastrophic insult; the remaining survivors usually evolve to a permanent vegetative or minimally conscious state.

TABLE 5-4. *Initial EEG findings in children with brain death*

Study	No. of patients	Percentage of patients with ECS
Green and Lauber, 1972 (40)	2	100%
Ashwal et al., 1977	11	82%
Holzman et al., 1983 (57)	18	61%
McMenamin and Volpe, 1983 (64)	3	100%
Furgiuele et al., 1984	10	91%
Coker and Dillehay, 1986 (55)	11	100%
Drake et al., 1986 (18)	47	70%
Ashwal et al., 1987 (5,6)	6	100%
Alvarez et al., 1988 (8)	52	100%
LaMancusa et al., 1991 (44)	92	100%
Parker et al., 1995 (2)	9	100%
Ashwal, 1997 (15)	37	51%
Ruiz-Lopez et al. 1999 (96)	29	48%
	332 (total)	83% (average)

ECS, electroencephalographic silence.

The Ad Hoc Task Force of the American Academy of Pediatrics recommends two EEGs in children below 1 year of age, but overall, the available data in children may suggest that documentation of isoelectric EEG on the initial recording is probably sufficient to support the clinical diagnosis of brain death (15). In addition, it is not necessary to obtain an EEG in children over 1 year of age as long as the neurologic examination remains unchanged for the appropriate time period of observation (10).

Electroencephalography may be confounded by hypothermia and drugs, and recordings in these circumstances unreliable. In children, suppression of EEG activity does not appear until 24°C (75.2°F), and the appearance of an isoelectric EEG does not occur until the temperature is below 18°C (64.4°F) (42,43). Nonetheless due to their smaller body mass compared to the adult, it is easier to control an infant's or child's body temperature with the use of heating lamps or mattresses.

In children, the most common medications causing the reversible loss of brain electrocortical activity include barbiturates, benzodiazepines, narcotics and certain intravenous (thiopental, ketamine, midazolam) and inhalation (halothane and isoflurane) anesthetics. Phenobarbital is the most common drug responsible for reversible isoelectric EEG, as it is widely used for seizure control. In this setting, previous studies have suggested that phenobarbital levels more than 25 μg/mL might suppress EEG activity to the point of isoelectric recordings. Another study in 92 children reported data suggesting that therapeutic levels of phenobarbital (i.e., 15 to 40 μg/mL) do not affect the EEG (44). Correlation with other antiepileptic agents has not been reported. The exact threshold in children remains difficult to ascertain, but serum levels below 20 to 25 μg/mL are unlikely to cause ECS, affect apnea testing or the examination of brainstem reflexes (13). (For pentobarbital level in ICP treatment see Chapter 6.)

Cerebral Blood Flow Determination

Neuroimaging techniques can be used to document the absence of CBF and include cerebral angiography, radionuclide scanning, transcranial Doppler (TCD), computed tomography with contrast injection or xenon inhalation, digital subtraction angiography, single photon emission computed tomography (SPECT), and positron emission tomography (PET). Documentation of the absence of CBF is considered confirmatory of brain death, but as shown in Table 5-5, not all infants and children who are brain dead show absence of CBF or abnormal TCD velocity patterns. In this section, a detailed description of the available literature follows.

Radionuclide scanning remains the most widely used test in children because it is portable, valid, and convenient to perform. With most methods, circulation is assessed during an early "dynamic" phase and later by examining static images for cerebral uptake of the specific radionuclide (usually technetium-99m pertechnetate, Tc-99m glucoheptonate, or tc-99m DTPA). During the dynamic phase a bolus of the radionuclide is rapidly injected and isotopic cranial images are obtained. During the arterial phase, cerebral activity is detectable within several seconds and, from the time of peak cerebral activity, sagittal sinus activity is observed within 6 to 8 s (49).

TABLE 5-5. *Cerebral blood flow or velocity studies in children with brain death*

Study	No. of patients	Percentage of patients with no CBF
Radionuclide angiography		
Ashwal et al., 1977	11	91%
Ashwal and Schneider, 1979 (37)	5	100%
Holzman et al., 1983 (57)	18	56%
Schwartz et al., 1984 (54)	9	100%
Coker and Dillehay, 1986 (55)	55	96%
Drake et al., 1986 (18)	42	64%
Ashwal et al., 1989 (45)	9	100%
Singh et al., 1994	26	77%
Parker et al., 1995 (2)	30	87%
Ashwal, 1997 (15)	18	72%
Transcranial Doppler		
McMenamin and Volpe, 1983 (64)	6	100%
Furgiuele et al., 1984	11	100%
Ahmann et al., 1987 (65)[a]	32	59%
Bode et al., 1988 (71)	9	89%
Glasier et al., 1989 (72)	9	89%
Messer et al., 1990 (68)	11	100%
Jalili et al., 1994 (70)	7	71%
Qian et al., 1998 (66)	17	100%
Cerebral angiography		
Parvey and Gerald, 1976	4	100%
Schwartz et al., 1984 (54)	9	100%
Xenon computed tomography		
Ashwal et al., 1989 (45)	10	100%
	348 (total)	83% (average)

[a] In the study of Ahmann et al. (65), 19/23 infants >4 months of age showed characteristic TCD changes seen with brain death; the remaining nine infants were less than 4 months old, and none showed a typical response.

If activity is not detectable in this early phase, CBF is considered absent. Most tracers have a half-life of several hours, and therefore, the static phase of a radionuclide imaging study is performed later to image absence or presence of diffuse parenchymal isotopic uptake. Currently, most centers are using SPECT scanning with Tc-99m hexylmethylpropylene amineoxine (HMPAO) as the isotopic agent (46–56). This agent is more lipophilic, is not dependent on the quality of the bolus injection, and enables more precise static imaging of parenchymatous brain. With this technology, isotope can be injected in the ICU and later images obtained using a mobile camera or after transfer of the patient to the nuclear medicine department.

Multiple studies in adults and children have documented that radionuclide imaging is accurate and reproducible and it has been favorably compared with other methods of detecting the presence or absence of CBF (2,18,39,45,55–57).

The absence of CBF in brain death is due primarily to very low cerebral perfusion pressure [mean arterial pressure (MAP) − (intracranial pressure (ICP)] and secondarily to release of vasoconstrictors from vascular smooth muscle and brain parenchyma. In the majority of brain-dead children studied at Loma Linda University Children's

Hospital, cerebral perfusion pressure has been calculated below 20 to 30 mm Hg when CBF was absent. However, four of 24 brain-dead children with absent CBF and with ICP monitoring had persistently high cerebral perfusion pressures greater than 45 to 50 mm Hg (56). Holzman et al. observed the same phenomena in four patients, ages 8 months to 3 years (57). Such findings indicate that, although several mechanisms may be involved in the loss of CBF during brain death, the majority are due to markedly increased ICP (50).

Some concern about specificity of the radionuclide imaging technique in newborns has been raised. Reduced CBF has been reported in preterm and term infants who survived with relatively intact neurologic function. For example, in one series of preterm infants, xenon cerebral flow values averaged 12 mL/min/100 g in 24 of 42 infants (58); in another small study of preterm infants using positron emission tomography (PET), flow values ranged from 7 to 11 mL/min/100 g (59). None of these patients were clinically brain dead.

In a study of eight brain-dead adults using stable xenon computed tomography, cerebral blood flow (XeCTCBF) measured 1.6 ± 2.0 mL/min/100 g (60). In another study of nine clinically brain-dead children, 1 month to 11 years of age, CBF determined by stable XeCTCBF was compared to radionuclide imaging techniques (45). All patients showed no flow by radionuclide imaging and had XeCTCBF values of 1.29 ± 1.6 mL/min/100 g. Although none of these patients were preterm infants, three were 1 month, 7 weeks, and 3 months of age. Both the adult and pediatric XeCTCBF investigations showed that CBF at the time of brain death was less than 2 mL/min/100 g and that this value correlated with the absence of flow by radionuclide imaging (45,60). Therefore, it is likely that radionuclide imaging, available in most hospitals, is valid in newborns as well as older infants and children for determination of CBF.

Clinically brain-dead pediatric patients have been reported who have presence of CBF early after diagnosis (Table 5-5). In the studies reported by Drake et al., 15 of 47 children who were clinically brain dead had evidence of intact CBF as determined by radionuclide imaging (18). About two-thirds of the patients who were restudied showed loss of CBF, 2 to 3 days later. This occurred irrespective of whether these patients had an isoelectric EEG or some residual activity recorded at the time the first CBF study was performed. In a more recent report, five of 18 clinically brain-dead preterm and term infants had retained CBF (14). Greisen and Pryds also reported two suspected brain-dead newborn infants with ECS who had preserved CBF documented by xenon scanning (61). Even more complicating in these neonates, phenobarbital and diazepam had been administered and a phenobarbital serum level of 42 mg/dL was detected in one of these patients. They were subsequently taken off respiratory support and neuropathologic examination was consistent with diffuse neuronal necrosis and the clinical diagnosis of brain death. Another report of a clinically brain-dead 2-month-old child found persistence of CBF and normal glucose metabolism by PET despite an isoelectric EEG. Neuropathologic examination showed extensive necrosis that was believed to be present at the time the PET scan was done (62). Overall, it is clear that CBF may be present in infants and children who are clinically brain dead. Repeat CBF studies 24 to 48 h later will likely but not uniformly document the loss of CBF. These observations suggest a somehow gradual halting of blood flow due to gradual increase in intracranial pressure finally going beyond the arterial pressure. Moreover, compensatory resources are more substantial in infants who have the ability to expand the skull by separating the sutures.

TCD sonography has been advocated because it is a portable and noninvasive method to ascertain cerebral circulatory arrest (63–71). Changes noted on TCD in brain death include loss of diastolic flow, appearance of retrograde diastolic flow, and diminution of systolic flow, and in occasional instances, with earlier documentation of a TCD signal, the loss of any detectable flow.

McMenamin and Volpe reported six brain-dead infants, 28 to 40 weeks gestation, who had the characteristic progression of velocity changes as cerebral edema and ICP increased (64). ICP in four of six infants was elevated and EEGs in three infants showed ECS. Although cerebral angiography or radionuclide imaging were not performed to corroborate the Doppler results, postmortem examination revealed brain necrosis consistent with brain death. In other studies, 19 of 23 brain-dead children older than 4 months showed a characteristic velocity pattern with a single sharp systolic peak followed by a rapid negative deflection below baseline, sharply rebounding to forward flow in early to mid-diastole with gradual tapering at the end of diastole to or below baseline (65). Eight of the 19 patients with this pattern also demonstrated absent CBF by radionuclide angiography. Infants less than 4 months of age who were studied had atypical waveforms, suggesting that the pulsed Doppler technique in newborns might not be as reliable.

More recent studies found similar Doppler velocity changes in 11 comatose children who progressed to brain death (68). Other studies, however, have found limitations to this technique. In one report, only five of seven brain-dead patients had bilateral reversal of flow (implying increased cerebrovascular resistance and absent cerebral circulation) (70). Bode and colleagues examined nine brain-dead children and in eight typical findings were reported (71). However, one newborn showed normal systolic and end-diastolic CBF velocities for 2 days despite clinical and EEG signs of brain death. Others have also encountered individual cases that did not show similar progression as originally described (72). In one case study of a brain-dead infant due to SIDS, TCD sonography demonstrated nearly normal cerebral perfusion, which even increased day by day, notwithstanding the persistence of other signs of brain death (73). To complicate matters even further, one case report found similar patterns of reversal of diastolic flow in a 1-month-old infant with status epilepticus who recovered without sequelae (74). The comparatively poor specificity of TCD in diagnosis of brain death in children may be due to brain injuries not increasing ICP and vascular resistance (e.g., asphyxia).

Digital subtraction angiography (DSA) is another technique that has been used to assess the intracranial circulation. This technique can be performed intravenously (71) or by intraarterial injection (75). A small amount of nonionic contrast material is injected while digital subtraction imaging of the cerebral vasculature is done, similar to conventional cerebral angiography. This allows visualization of contrast within the major intracranial vessels; lack of such visualization indicates absence of CBF and, beyond question, brain death. There are very few reports of this technique in children and only one recent case report in a brain-dead neonate (76). A 1989 report using intravenous DSA in 110 patients aged 3 to 83 years with clinical signs of brain death observed absent contrast enhancement in 105 patients (75). Repeat studies in the remaining five patients within several hours confirmed the cessation of CBF.

Stable xenon and 133-xenon computed tomography are examples of useful, reliable, and well documented tests that are now seldom used due to cost, need for upgraded computer software programs and specially trained personnel (77). Xenon CT allows quantitative and regional measurement of CBF. In brain-dead adults, CBF values of 1.6 ± 2.0 mL/min/100 g have been reported (60). Previous studies found an average CBF of 1.3 ± 1.6 mL/min/100 g in 10 brain-dead children, substantially lower than when compared to CBF of 33.5 ± 16.3 mL/min/100 g in 11 profoundly comatose children (45). In addition, CBF studies were much higher in preterm infants who suffered neurologic injury but who were not brain dead. CBF values in these studies were 12 mL/min/100 g using 133-xenon (58) and 7 to 11 mL/min/100 g using PET scanning (59), but these values did not approximate those found in comatose infants with retained brainstem function.

The results of PET scanning have been reported in only a few brain-dead pediatric patients (62,78). Because of its limited availability, cost and lack of comparison studies, it offers no advantages to the more standardized methods previously discussed. Meyer reported an 18-year-old brain-dead adolescent whose dynamic PET study, performed 7 days after a severe traumatic closed-head injury, showed no intracerebral uptake or retention of tracer and was considered consistent with diffuse absence of brain metabolism (78). Medlock and colleagues reported a 2-month-old brain-dead infant with preserved CBF whose PET scan on the 11th day following injury showed a normal glucose metabolic gradient between gray and white matter (62). Autopsy revealed widespread necrosis with mononuclear cell infiltrates throughout the cerebral cortex. The persistence of glucose metabolism was thought to be associated with the presence of inflammatory microglial cells and suggested that persistence of CBF and glucose metabolism in brain-dead children might not reflect neuronal survival.

Magnetic resonance imaging (MRI) has been reported in small series of adult brain-dead patients (79–82). Characteristic features are described and illustrated in Chapter 4, but have not been confirmed in children.

In the past two decades phosphorus (^{31}P) and proton (^{1}H) magnetic resonance spectroscopy (MRS) have been used to noninvasively measure aspects of brain metabolic activity. Recent studies in the neonate and in older infants and children have shown significant abnormalities using these techniques documenting loss of metabolic activity associated with severe acute central nervous system insults (83,84). Kato et al. reported ^{31}P-MRS in three infants, four children, and 17 adults who were clinically brain dead. Spectra demonstrated the absence of adenosine triphosphate (ATP) and phosphocreatine (PCr) while the inorganic phosphate and phosphodiesterase peaks were still detectable (85). Another ^{31}P-MRS study involving three brain-dead adults found similar spectral abnormalities (86). These findings suggest that MRS could provide another technique to objectively assess the complete loss of cerebral function. The advantage of MRS is that it can be done in conjunction with MRI. This allows acquisition of anatomic as well as metabolic data that could further clarify the etiology of the CNS insult and at the same time determine whether there is irreversible neuronal loss. Representative of the often repeated theme of conflicting reports, Terk and coinvestigators reported a term brain-dead infant whose ^{31}P spectra on days 11 and 18 demonstrated three distinct ATP peaks as well as several other peaks that suggested the persistence of metabolic activity (87). Although no definite reasons could be ascertained for this finding compared to the study of Kato and colleagues (85), Terk and colleagues suggested that any proposed spectral signature for brain death would need to be modified (87).

There are no published case reports concerning proton MRS and brain death in children. Recently at Loma Linda University Children's Hospital seven brain-dead children were studied with proton MRS. All spectra were markedly abnormal with severe reductions or loss of the metabolite peaks (*N*-acetylaspartate, choline, creatine) and a clearly identifiable and elevated lactate peak. Review of these findings compared to other children who were severely brain injured but not brain dead did not demonstrate any obvious differences although it appeared that the reductions in the *N*-acetylaspartate peak were markedly reduced to absent in the gray matter spectra (Fig. 5-2), whereas it was still discernible in the white matter (Fig. 5-3).

Evoked Responses

Brainstem auditory evoked response (BAER) testing has been extensively studied as an alternative confirmatory method (88–92). Several studies have raised doubt as to its value in brain death determination, particularly in children less than 6 months of age (88,92–95) but more recent studies claim that BAER is reliable (96,97). In one report, 90% of 51 brain-dead children had loss of the BAER (complete loss in 27 patients; loss of waveforms III to VII in 18 patients) (96). It was also shown that loss of the BAER preceded flattening of the EEG. This finding suggested that BAER testing might be more useful than the EEG for earlier laboratory confirmation of brain death. However, if BAER testing is performed too "early," a false positive test may result. In one recent report, return of an absent BAER was observed in a 28-month-old infant 18 h after a severe global hypoxic-ischemic insult (41).

It is doubtful whether somatosensory evoked potentials (SSEPs) have greater discrimination in the confirmation of brain death (97–102). Recent SSEP studies in children found that only 62.5% of patients had the complete absence of the summated response or only a cervical cord response suggesting limitation of SSEPs as a confirmatory test in children (92). In addition, absent evoked potentials may be observed in other comatose states.

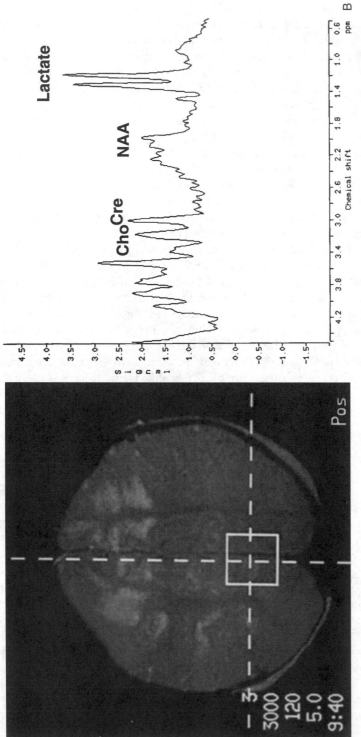

FIG. 5-2. Proton magnetic resonance (MR) spectroscopy in 3-month-old boy who was brain dead after suspected nonaccidental trauma. **A:** Axial T2-weighted spin-echo image obtained 1 day after admission shows edema and swelling of cortical and subcortical vascular border zones. Increased signal intensity was also noted in the right basal ganglia consistent with a history of acute cerebral anoxia. A highlighted box shows the $2 \times 2 \times 2$ cm³ volume in occipital gray matter in which the proton spectrum is acquired. **B:** Proton MR spectrum (TR/TE = 3,000/20 ms, stimulated echo acquisition mode) obtained immediately after imaging shows a prominent lactate (Lac) peak. The NAA/Cre ratio is decreased by 75% and the NAA/Cho ratio is decreased by 50% compared to age-matched control values. (Courtesy of Dr. Barbara Holshouser, Department of Radiology, Loma Linda University Children's Hospital.)

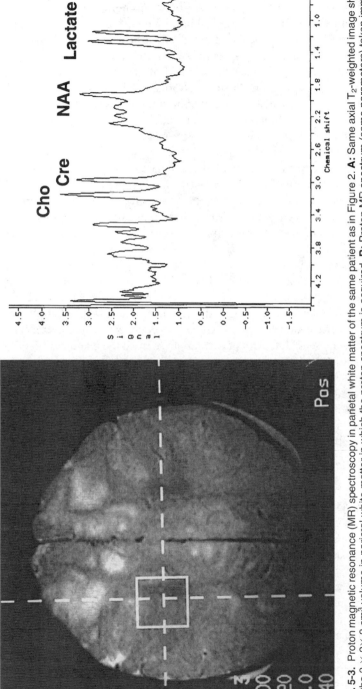

FIG. 5-3. Proton magnetic resonance (MR) spectroscopy in parietal white matter of the same patient as in Figure 2. **A:** Same axial T₂-weighted image showing the 2 × 2 × 2 cm³ volume in parietal white matter in which the proton spectrum is acquired. **B:** Proton MR spectrum (same parameters) taken immediately after the above spectrum also shows a prominent lactate (Lac) peak and decreased NAA/Cre and NAA/Cho ratios. Although significantly decreased compared to normal values, the NAA level in white matter was found to be higher than in the same volume of occipital gray matter. (Courtesy of Dr. Barbara Holshouser, Department of Radiology, Loma Linda University Children's Hospital).

BRAIN DEATH IN NEWBORNS

A recent review estimates that each year about 550 newborns out of a total of 4,900,000 live births might be diagnosed as brain dead (15). Etiologies of brain death based on data from 87 newborns less than 1 month of age included hypoxic-ischemic encephalopathy (61%), birth trauma (8%), malformations (6%), cerebral hemorrhage (6%), infection (7%), SIDS (7%), nonaccidental trauma (4%), and metabolic causes (1%).

The ability to diagnose brain death in newborns is still viewed with uncertainty (15). This is due primarily to the small number of brain-dead neonates reported in the literature. Preterm and term neonates less than 7 days of age were excluded from the 1987 pediatric brain death guidelines. It was phrased as follows: "The newborn is difficult to evaluate clinically after perinatal insults. This relates to many factors including difficulties of clinical assessment, determination of proximate cause of coma, and certainty of the validity of laboratory tests. These problems are accentuated in a premature infant" (10). Several years after the publication of these guidelines, data on 18 brain-dead neonates were published and it was suggested that brain death could be diagnosed in term infants and preterm infants greater than 34 weeks gestational age within the first week of life (14). Because the newborn has patent sutures and an open fontanel, increases in ICP after acute injury are not as significant as in older patients. Thus, the usual cascade of events of herniation that results from increased ICP and reduced cerebral perfusion are less likely to occur in the newborn. Brain death in the newborn can be diagnosed providing the physician is aware of the limitations of the clinical examination and laboratory testing. It is important to carefully and repeatedly examine these infants with particular attention to the examination of brainstem reflexes and apnea testing.

Specific issues regarding certainty of diagnosis, immaturity of the nervous system, and the effects of development on the pathophysiology and diagnosis of brain death in the preterm and term infant have also previously been published (34,103–105) and recently updated (15). For the most part, Task Force recommendations concerning the duration of observation of brain death in infants and children of different ages were based on expert opinion and consensus rather than evidence based. Recently collected data from 87 newborns allowed the following estimations: (a) the duration of coma from impact to brain death (37 h); (b) duration of time before brain death confirmation (75 h); and (c) the duration of time to transplantation (20 h) (15). The average duration of brain death in these patients was about 95 h (or almost 4 days). In none of the patients was recovery of brainstem function observed. The duration of brain death was also specifically analyzed in 53 neonates donating organs for transplantation. The total duration of brain death (including time to transplantation) averaged 2.8 days in neonates less than 7 days of age. In the neonates 1 to 3 weeks of age, the duration of brain death was approximately 5.2 days. The data suggest that a 24- to 48-h period of observation in neonates, even in those less than 7 days of age, should be sufficient to establish the diagnosis of brain death.

Because of the significant pathophysiologic differences in the neonatal response to injuries resulting in brain death, previous studies have observed a much higher incidence of newborns with EEG activity or cerebral perfusion (15). In addition, some newborns with isoelectric EEGs showed preserved CBF and, conversely, others without CBF showed EEG activity. In the neonate, even though CBF and mean arterial blood pressures are much lower, increases in ICP after acute injury are less dramatic. Recent data on 30 newborns who had EEGs and radionuclide perfusion studies found that one-third with isoelectric EEG showed evidence of CBF and 58% of those with absent CBF had evidence of EEG activity (15).

Data on 37 of 53 brain-dead newborns in whom EEGs were performed revealed the following: isoelectric recording ($n = 21$); very-low-voltage ($n = 13$); burst-suppression ($n = 1$); seizure activity ($n = 1$); normal ($n = 1$) (15). Almost all patients whose first EEG showed ECS had ECS on the second study and most of the patients who initially did not show ECS on their first EEG did so on a repeat study. The data suggest that for confirmation of brain death only one isoelectric EEG is necessary, providing the examination over a fixed time interval remains unchanged.

In a 1989 review on neonatal brain death, CBF data were reported in 29 patients (14). One infant had contrast cerebral angiography, nine had Doppler and 19 had radionuclide isotopic scans. The outcome of the 11 patients without radionuclide uptake included cardiac arrest ($n = 3$), discontinuation of respiratory support an average of 5 days after diagnosis ($n = 7$), and short-term survival ($n = 1$). Almost one-third of the infants in that study who had radionuclide scans had evidence of cerebral perfusion.

CBF data are now available on an additional 18 patients taken from a larger retrospective review of neonatal brain death reported in 1997 (15). In 72% of these infants CBF was not detected. The median duration of brain death in these 13 patients was 4 days, with four patients showing isoelectric EEG and four patients with low-voltage slow-wave activity. Of the five neonates with CBF, only two had repeat studies and in one CBF was still present. This infant initially had a normal EEG but two follow-up studies showed isoelectric EEG. No significant differences were noted in the median duration of brain death in those neonates with CBF (4 days) compared to those without CBF (3 days). These findings as well as those described earlier again emphasize the limitations of both CBF determinations and EEG findings for brain death confirmation in neonates. To epitomize, an observation period of 48 h is recommended to confirm the diagnosis. If an EEG is isoelectric or if a CBF study shows no flow, the observation period can be shortened to 24 h. Although there are few cases of preterm infants who are brain dead, it is likely that the same time frame would be applicable. There have been few instances of neonates or older infants who showed minimal transient clinical or EEG recovery but none appear to have regained meaningful neurologic function and all died within brief periods of time.

BRAIN DEATH IN INFANTS WITH ANENCEPHALY

Infants with anencephaly have been considered as possible sources for organ donation but have generated considerable controversy (106–109). This again drew widespread media attention when the American Medical Association Council report (that was subsequently rescinded) recommended that liveborn anencephalic infants, who did not meet accepted brain death criteria, could be considered for organ donation (106,108). Because anencephalic infants demonstrate brainstem function, they do not meet the legal requirements of whole brain death as called for by the Uniform Determination of Death Act.

Diagnosis of brain death in anencephalic infants requires careful evaluation because of the severe central nervous system malformations that are present, particularly in the brainstem (108). However, brain death can be diagnosed by specifically determining the absence or loss of preexisting brainstem function including apnea. Difficulties in performing the examination have been previously reviewed (108). Serial examinations demonstrating the loss of any previously detectable cranial nerve reflexes and the performance of repeated apnea challenge studies documenting the absence of respiratory effort with a $Paco_2$ greater than 60 mm Hg over 24 to 48 h should be considered in keeping with previously published guidelines on brain death. It is recommended that the period of observation to confirm the diagnosis of brain death be similar, that is, 24 to 48 h.

FETAL BRAIN DEATH

Fetal brain death is recognized by the presence of a prolonged fixed fetal heart rate pattern (even following different types of stress tests); an atonic fetus without breathing and body movement; the appearance of polyhydramnios; and the development of ventriculomegaly (110,111). The first case, after an uncomplicated pregnancy, was reported in 1977 on the basis of clinical criteria of neonatal brain death with neuropathologic evidence of diffuse central nervous system destruction typical of severe intrauterine anoxia and circulatory failure (112). Fetal brain death during pregnancy is an extremely rare event with probably less than 20 patients reported (110,113).

ORGAN PROCUREMENT IN BRAIN-DEAD CHILDREN

Because brain death is more frequently due to severe asphyxial injury in children than in adults, a risk exists that similar injury to other organs may preclude transplantation. Inotropic agents to support blood pressure and cardiac function are necessary, particularly if the etiology of brain death was related to a preexisting global asphyxial insult which may have caused hypoxic myocardial injury (114). Organ transplantation can be successfully accomplished from pediatric donors (115). Brain-dead child abuse victims have infrequently been considered organ donors due to legal issues, but many centers have now tried to obtain surrogate consent and with cooperation from the medical examiner's office have been able to successfully harvest organs (116). The principles of management of the brain-dead child are comparable to those in adults and discussed in Chapter 10.

CONCLUSION

It is expected that a certain percentage of infants and children, much like adults, will have neurodiagnostic testing results that do not fit the clinical examination. As is the case in many other areas of pediatrics, serial examinations should allow for the establishment of a definitive diagnosis. Better understanding of the pathophysiology of the evolution of brain death in neonates and infants should help decide whether recommended age-related periods of observation are justified.

REFERENCES

1. Ryan CA, Byrne P, Kuhn S, et al. No resuscitation and withdrawal of therapy in a neonatal and a pediatric intensive care unit in Canada. *J Pediatr* 1993;123:534–538.
2. Parker BL, Frewen TC, Levin SD, et al. Declaring pediatric brain death: current practice in a Canadian pediatric critical care unit. *Can Med Assoc J* 1995;153:909–916.
3. Mejia RE, Pollack MM. Variability in brain death determination practices in children. *JAMA* 1995; 274:550–553.
4. Martinot A, Lejeune C, Hue V, et al. Modality and causes of 259 deaths in a pediatric intensive care unit. *Arch Pediatr* 1995;2:735–741.
5. Ashwal S, Schneider S. Brain death in children: Part I. *Pediatr Neurol* 1987;3:5–10.
6. Ashwal S, Schneider S. Brain death in children: Part II. *Pediatr Neurol* 1987;3:9–77.
7. Rowland RW, Donnelly JH, Jackson AH, et al. Brain death in the pediatric intensive care unit. *Am J Dis Child* 1983;137:547–550.
8. Alvarez LA, Moshe SL, Belman AL, et al. EEG and brain death determination in children. *Neurology* 1988;38:227–230.
9. Wijdicks EFM. Determining brain death in adults. *Neurology* 1995;45:1003–1011.
10. Guidelines for the determination of brain death in children. *Pediatrics* 1987;80:298–300.
11. Kaufman HH, ed. *Pediatric brain death and organ/tissue retrieval: medical, ethical, and legal aspects.* New York: Plenum, 1989.
12. Farrell MM, Levin DL. Brain death in the pediatric patient: historical, sociological, medical, religious, cultural, legal, and ethical considerations. *Crit Care Med* 1993;21:1951–1965.
13. Ashwal S. Brain death in early infancy. *J Heart Lung Transplant* 1993;12:S176–S178.
14. Ashwal S, Schneider S. Brain death in the newborn. Clinical, EEG and blood flow determinations. *Pediatrics* 1989;84:429–437.
15. Ashwal S. Brain death in the newborn. Current perspectives. *Clin Perinatol* 1997;24:859–882.
16. Harrison AM, Botkin JR. Can pediatricians define and apply the concept of brain death? *Pediatrics* 1999;103:e82.
17. Lynch J, Eldadah MK. Brain-death criteria currently used by pediatric intensivists. *Clin Pediatr* 1992;31:457–460.
18. Drake B, Ashwal S, Schneider S. Determination of cerebral death in the pediatric intensive care unit. *Pediatrics* 1986;78:107–112.
19. Ashwal S. The persistent vegetative state in children. *Adv Pediatr* 1994;41:195–222.
20. Fanaroff A, Martin RJ, Miller MJ. The respiratory system. In: Fanaroff A, Martin RJ, eds. *Neonatal-perinatal medicine: diseases of the fetus and newborn.* St. Louis: CV Mosby, 1987:617.
21. Hack M. The sensorimotor development of the preterm infant. In: Fanaroff A, Martin RJ, eds. *Neonatal-perinatal medicine: diseases of the fetus and newborn.* St. Louis: CV Mosby, 1987:473.
22. Swaiman KF. Neurological examination of the preterm infant. In: Swaiman KF, ed. *Pediatric neurology: principles and practice.* St. Louis: Mosby, 1994:61.
23. Rowland TW, Donnelly JH, Jackson AH. Apnea documentation for determination of brain death in children. *Pediatrics* 1984;74:505–508.
24. Outwater KM, Rockoff MA. Apnea testing to confirm brain death in children. *Crit Care Med* 1984; 12:357–358.
25. Paret G, Barzilay Z. Apnea testing in suspected brain dead children–physiological and mathematical modeling. *Intensive Care Med* 1995;21:247–252.
26. Ammar A, Awada A, Al-Luwami I. Reversibility of severe brain stem dysfunction in children. *Acta Neurochir* 1993;124:86–91.
27. Okamoto K, Sugimoto T. Return of spontaneous respiration in an infant who fulfilled current criteria to determine brain death. *Pediatrics* 1995;96:518–520.
28. Fishman MA. Validity of brain death criteria in infants. *Pediatrics* 1995;96:513–515.
29. Vardis R, Pollack MM. Increased apnea threshold in a pediatric patient with suspected brain death. *Crit Care Med* 1998;26:1917–1919.

30. American Electroencephalographic Society. Guideline three: minimum technical standards for EEG recording in suspected cerebral death. *J Clin Neurophysiol* 1994;11:10–13.
31. Kohrman MH, Spivack BS. Brain death in infants: sensitivity and specificity of current criteria. *Pediatr Neurol* 1990;6:47–50.
32. Moshe S. Usefulness of EEG in the evaluation of brain death in children: the pros. *Electroencephalogr Clin Neurophysiol* 1989;73:272–275.
33. Schneider S. Usefulness of EEG in the evaluation of brain death in children: the cons. *Electroencephalogr Clin Neurophysiol* 1989;73:276–278.
34. Ashwal S. Brain death in the newborn. *Clin Perinatol* 1989;16:501–518.
35. Volpe JJ. Commentary—brain death determination in the newborn. *Pediatrics* 1987;80:293–297.
36. Ashwal S, Schneider S. Pediatric brain death: current perspectives. In: Barness LA, ed. *Advances in pediatrics. Volume 38.* Chicago: Mosby Year Book, 1991:181–202.
37. Ashwal S, Schneider S. Failure of electroencephalography to diagnose brain death in comatose patients. *Ann Neurol* 1979;6:512–517.
38. Grigg G, Kelly M, Celesia G, et al. Electroencephalographic activity after brain death. *Arch Neurol* 1987;44:948–954.
39. Ruiz-Garcia M, Gonzalez-Astiazaran A, Collado-Corona MA, et al. Brain death in children: clinical, neurophysiological and radioisotopic angiography findings in 125 patients. *Childs Nerv Syst* 2000; 16:40–46.
40. Green JR, Lauber A. Recovery of activity in young children after ECS. *J Neurol Neurosurg Psychiatry* 1972;35:103–107.
41. Schmitt B, Simma B, Burger R, et al. Resuscitation after severe hypoxia in a young child: temporary isoelectric EEG and loss of BAEP components. *Intensive Care Med* 1993;19:420–422.
42. Hicks RC, Poole JL. Electroencephalographic changes with hypothermia and cardiopulmonary bypass in children. *J Thorac Cardiovasc Surg* 1981;81:781–786.
43. Jorgensen EO, Malchow-Moller A. Cerebral prognostic signs during cardiopulmonary resuscitation. *Resuscitation* 1978;6:217–225.
44. LaMancusa J, Cooper R, Vieth R, et al. The effects of the falling therapeutic and subtherapeutic barbiturate blood levels on electrocerebral silence in clinically brain-dead children. *Clin Electroencephalogr* 1991;22:112–117.
45. Ashwal S, Schneider S, Thompson J. Xenon computed tomography measuring cerebral blood flow in the determination of brain death in children. *Ann Neurol* 1989;25:539–546.
46. Mrhac L, Zakko S, Parikh Y. Brain death: the evaluation of semi-quantitative parameters and other signs in HMPAO scintigraphy. *Nucl Med Commun* 1995;16:1016–1020.
47. Wilson K, Gormon L, Seeby JB. The diagnosis of brain death with Tc-99m HmPAO. *Clin Nucl Med* 1993;18:428–434.
48. Bonetti MG, Ciritella P, Valle G, et al. ^{99m}Tc HM-PAO brain perfusion SPECT in brain death. *Neuroradiology* 1995;37:365–369.
49. Wieler H, March K, Kaisar KP, et al. Tc-99m HMPAO cerebral scintigraphy: a reliable, noninvasive method for determination of brain death. *Clin Nucl Med* 1993;18:104–109.
50. Villani A, Onofri A, Bianchi R, et al. Determination of brain death in intensive pediatric therapy. *Pediatr Med Chir* 1998;20:19–23.
51. Valle G, Ciritella P, Bonetti MG, et al. Considerations of brain death on a SPECT cerebral perfusion study. *Clin Nucl Med* 1993;18:953–954.
52. Abdel Dayem HM, Bahar RH, Sigurdsson GH, et al. The hollow skull: a sign of brain death in Tc-99m HM-PAO brain scintigraphy. *Clin Nucl Med* 1989;14:912–916.
53. Galaske RG, Schober O, Heyer R. ^{99m}Tc-HM-PAO and ^{123}I-amphetamine cerebral scintigraphy: a new, non-invasive method in determination of brain death in children. *Eur J Nucl Med* 1988; 14:446–452.
54. Schwartz JA, Baxter J, Brill DR. Diagnosis of brain death in children by radionuclide cerebral imaging. *Pediatrics* 1984;73:14–18.
55. Coker SB, Dillehay GL. Radionuclide cerebral imaging for confirmation of brain death in children: the significance of dural sinus activity. *Pediatr Neurol* 1986;2:43–46.
56. Goodman JM, Heck LL, Moore BD. Confirmation of brain death with portable isotope angiography: a review of 204 consecutive cases. *Neurosurgery* 1985;16:492–497.
57. Holzman BH, Curless RG, Sfakianakis GN, et al. Radionuclide cerebral perfusion scintigraphy in determination of brain death in children. *Neurology* 1983;33:1027–1031.
58. Greisen G. Cerebral blood flow in preterm infants during the first week of life. *Acta Paediatr Scand* 1986;75:43–51.

59. Altman DL, Powers WJ, Perlman JM, et al. Cerebral blood flow requirements for brain viability in newborn infants is lower than in adults. *Ann Neurol* 1988;24:218–226.
60. Darby JM, Yonas H, Gur D, et al. Xenon-enhanced computed tomography in brain death. *Arch Neurol* 1987;44:551–554.
61. Greisen G, Pryds O, Low CBF. Discontinuous EEG activity, and periventricular brain injury in ill, preterm neonates. *Brain Dev* 1989;11:164–168
62. Medlock MD, Hanigan WC, Cruse RP. Dissociation of cerebral blood flow, glucose metabolism, and electrical activity in pediatric brain death. *J Neurosurg* 1993;79:752–775.
63. Ducrocq X, Hassler W, Moritake K, et al. Consensus opinion on diagnosis of cerebral circulatory arrest using Doppler-sonography: Task Force Group on Cerebral Death of the Neurosonology Research Group of the World Federation of Neurology. *J Neurol Sci* 1998;159:145–150.
64. McMenamin JB, Volpe JJ. Doppler ultrasonography in the determination of neonatal brain death. *Ann Neurol* 1983;14:302–307.
65. Ahmann PA, Carrigan TA, Carlton D, et al. Brain death in children. Characteristic common carotid arterial velocity patterns measured with pulsed Doppler ultrasound. *J Pediatr* 1987;110:723–728.
66. Qian SY, Fan XM, Yin HH. Transcranial Doppler assessment of brain death in children. *Singapore Med J* 1998;39:247–250.
67. Feri M, Ralli L, Felici M, et al. Transcranial Doppler and brain death diagnosis. *Crit Care Med* 1994; 22:1120–1126.
68. Messer J, Burtscher A, Haddad J, et al. Contribution of transcranial Doppler sonography to the diagnosis of brain death in children. *Arch Fr Pediatr* 1990;47:647–651.
69. Manno EM. Transcranial Doppler ultrasonography in the neurocritical care unit. *Crit Care Clin* 1997;13:79–104.
70. Jalili M, Crade M, Davis AL. Carotid blood-flow velocity changes detected by Doppler ultrasound in determination of brain death in children. A preliminary report. *Clin Pediatr Phila* 1994; 33:669–674.
71. Bode H, Sauer M, Pringsheim W. Diagnosis of brain death by transcranial Doppler sonography. *Arch Dis Child* 1988;63:1474–1478.
72. Glasier CM, Seibert JJ, Chadduck WM, et al. Brain death in infants: evaluation with Doppler US. *Radiology* 1989;172:377–380.
73. Sanker P, Roth B, Frowein RA, et al. Cerebral reperfusion in brain death of a newborn. Case report. *Neurosurg Rev* 1992;15:315–317.
74. Chiu NC, Shen EY, Lee BS. Reversal of diastolic cerebral blood flow in infants without brain death. *Pediatr Neurol* 1994;11:337–340.
75. Van Bunnen Y, Delcour C, Wery D, et al. Intravenous digital subtraction angiography. A criteria of brain death. *Ann Radiol (Paris)* 1989;32:279–281.
76. Albertini A, Schonfeld S, Hiatt M, et al. Digital subtraction angiography—a new approach to brain death determination in the newborn. *Pediatr Radiol* 1993;23:195–197.
77. Pistoia F, Johnson DW, Darby JM, et al. The role of xenon CT measurements of cerebral blood flow in the clinical determination of brain death. *AJNR Am J Neuroradiol* 1991;12:97–103.
78. Meyer MA. Evaluating brain death with positron emission tomography: case report on dynamic imaging of ^{18}F-fluorodeoxyglucose activity after intravenous bolus injection. *J Neuroimaging* 1996; 6:117–119.
79. Orrison WW Jr, Champlin AM, Kesterson OL, et al. MR "hot nose sign" and "intravascular enhancement sign" in brain death. *AJNR Am J Neuroradiol* 1994;15:913–916.
80. Lee DH, Nathanson JA, Fox AJ, et al. Magnetic resonance imaging of brain death. *Can Assoc Radiol J* 1995;46:174–178.
81. Matsumura A, Meguro K, Tsurushima H, et al. Magnetic resonance imaging of brain death. *Neurol Med Chir (Tokyo)* 1996;36:166–171.
82. Ishii K, Onuma T, Kinoshita T, et al. Brain death: MR and MR angiography. *AJNR Am J Neuroradiol* 1996;17:731–735.
83. Holshouser BA, Ashwal S, Luh GY, et al. Proton MR spectroscopy after acute central nervous system injury: outcome prediction in neonates, infants and children. *Radiology* 1997;202:487–496.
84. Martin E, Buchli R, Ritter S, et al. Diagnostic and prognostic value of cerebral ^{31}P magnetic resonance spectroscopy in neonates with perinatal asphyxia. *Pediatr Res* 1996;40:749–758.
85. Kato T, Tokumaru A, O'uchi T, et al. Assessment of brain death in children by means of P-31 MR spectroscopy: preliminary note. *Radiology* 1991;179:95–99.
86. Aichner F, Felber S, Birbamer G, et al. Magnetic resonance: a noninvasive approach to metabolism, circulation, and morphology in human brain death. *Ann Neurol* 1992;32:507–511.

87. Terk MR, Gober JR, DeGiorgio C, et al. Brain death in the neonate: assessment with P-31 MR spectroscopy. *Radiology* 1992;182:582–583.
88. Guerit JM. Evoked potentials: a safe brain-death confirmatory tool? *Eur J Med* 1992;1:233–243.
89. Machado C, Valdes P, Garcia Tigera J, et al. Brain-stem auditory evoked potentials and brain death. *Electroencephalogr Clin Neurophysiol* 1991;80:392–398.
90. Lutschg J, Pfenninger J, Ludin HP, et al. Brain-stem auditory evoked potentials and early somatosensory evoked potentials in neurointensively treated comatose children. *Am J Dis Child* 1983; 137:421–426.
91. Litscher G, Schwartz G, Kleinert R. Brainstem auditory evoked potential monitoring. Variations of stimulus artifact in brain death. *Electroencephalogr Clin Neurophysiol* 1995;96:413–419.
92. Steinhart CM, Weiss IP. Use of brainstem auditory evoked potentials in pediatric brain death. *Crit Care Med* 1985;13:560–562.
93. Taylor MJ, Houston BD, Lowry NJ. Recovery of auditory brainstem responses after a severe hypoxic ischemic insult. *N Engl J Med* 1983;309:1169–1170.
94. Dear PRF, Godfrey DJ. Neonatal auditory brainstem response cannot reliably diagnose brainstem death. *Arch Dis Child* 1985;60:17–19.
95. De Meirleir LJ, Taylor MJ. Evoked potentials in comatose children. Auditory brain stem responses. *Pediatr Neurol* 1986;2:31–34.
96. Ruiz-Lopez MJ, Martinez de Azagra A, Serrano A, et al. Brain death and evoked potentials in pediatric patients. *Crit Care Med* 1999;27:412–416.
97. Butinar D, Gostisa A. Brainstem auditory evoked potentials and somatosensory evoked potentials in prediction of posttraumatic coma in children. *Pflugers Arch* 1996;431:R289–R290.
98. Beca J, Cox PN, Taylor MJ, et al. Somatosensory evoked potentials for prediction of outcome in acute severe brain injury. *J Pediatr* 1995;126:44–49.
99. Wagner W. Scalp, earlobe and nasopharyngeal recordings of the median nerve somatosensory evoked p14 potential in coma and brain death. Detailed latency and amplitude analysis in 181 patients. *Brain* 1996;119:1507–1521.
100. Machado C. Multimodality evoked potentials and electroretinography in a test battery for an early diagnosis of brain death. *J Neurosurg Sci* 1993;37:125–131.
101. Goldie WD, Chiappa KH, Young RR, et al. Brainstem auditory and short-latency somatosensory evoked responses in brain death. *Neurology* 1981;31:248–256.
102. Facco E, Casartelli Liviero M, Munari M, et al. Short latency evoked potentials: new criteria for brain death? *J Neurol Neurosurg Psychiatry* 1990;53:351–353.
103. Kohrman MH. Brain death in neonates. *Semin Neurol* 1993;13:116–122.
104. Freeman JM, Ferry PC. New brain death guidelines in children: further confusion. *Pediatrics* 1988; 81:301–303.
105. Coulter DL. Neurologic uncertainty in newborn intensive care. *N Engl J Med* 1987;316:840–844.
106. American Medical Association. Council on Ethical and Judicial Affairs. The use of anencephalic neonates as organ donors. *JAMA* 1995;273:1614–1618.
107. The Medical Task Force on Anencephaly: the infant with anencephaly. *N Engl J Med* 1990; 22:669–674.
108. Walters J, Ashwal S, Masek T. Anencephaly: where do we now stand? *Semin Neurol* 1997; 17:249–255.
109. Ashwal S, Peabody JL, Schneider S, et al. Anencephaly: clinical determination of brain death and neuropathologic studies. *Pediatr Neurol* 1990;6:233–239.
110. Zimmer EZ, Jakobi P, Goldstein I, et al. Cardiotocographic and sonographic findings in two cases of antenatally diagnosed intrauterine fetal brain death. *Prenat Diagn* 1992;12:271–276.
111. Nijhuis JG, Crevels AJ, van Dongen PW. Fetal brain death: the definition of a fetal heart rate pattern and its clinical consequences. *Obstet Gynecol Surv* 1990;45:229–232.
112. Adams RD, Prod'hom LS, Rabinowicz T. Intrauterine brain death. Neuraxial reticular core necrosis. *Acta Neuropathol (Berl)* 1977;40:41–49.
113. James SJ. Fetal brain death syndrome—a case report and literature review. *Aust N Z J Obstet Gynaecol* 1998;38:217–220.
114. Goldstein B, DeKing D, DeLong DJ, et al. Autonomic cardiovascular state after severe brain injury and brain death in children. *Crit Care Med* 1993;21:228–233.
115. Doroshow RW, Ashwal S, Saukel GW. Availability and selection of donors for pediatric heart transplantation. *J Heart Lung Transplant* 1995;14:52–58.
116. Duthie SE, Peterson BM, Cutler J, et al. Successful organ donation in victims of child abuse. *Clin Transplant* 1995;9:415–418.

6

Neurologic States Resembling Brain Death

Eelco F. M. Wijdicks

Department of Neurology, Mayo Clinic, Rochester, Minnesota

In a monograph on brain death, it is fitting to discuss other neurologic conditions that can mimic brain death or are related to brain death in some measure. Relevant to clinical practice are comatose states that completely mimic structural damage to the brain (such as poisoning or hypothermia), comatose states that are due to catastrophic damage but have not entirely progressed to brain death, and neurologic conditions that have been confused with brain death but, in a sense, at least for neurologists, by no means resemble brain death (such as locked-in syndrome or vegetative state).

As stated in Chapter 4, there is no evidence of a disturbing trend in the clinical assessment of brain death, although occasionally cases of errors by physicians give notice (1). Usually, these cases contain very little neurologic detail and are typically reported in a journalistic fashion. However, one frequently quoted study, a survey among health professionals, found major differences in assessment of brain death and vegetative state among respondents when two fictitious cases were presented. This study, by Youngner et al. (2), included intensive care nurses, medical residents, attending anesthesiologists, operating room nurses, and intensive-care-unit physicians, but only a handful of attending and resident neurosurgeons and no neurologists. This particular study claimed that two-thirds of the physicians were unable to correctly identify or apply the criteria for the determination of brain death and, equally relevant, had difficulty distinguishing brain death from persistent vegetative state.

Neurologic states that should be set apart from brain death are presented, along with ways to prevent mistaken interpretation. It is beyond the scope of this monograph to present an exhaustive discussion of all toxins and poisons, and major handbooks should be reviewed as well.

MIMICKING DISORDERS

This section discusses disorders that closely (but often not completely) mimic brain death. These conditions should be excluded before any clinical evaluation of a patient with possible brain death is initiated.

Hypothermia

The anterior hypothalamus is the main regulating center involved in keeping a consistent core temperature of 36°C to 37.5°C. Hypothermia is defined as a core temperature of 35°C or less (3). The degrees of hypothermia have been arbitrarily categorized (Table 6-1). The effect of hypothermia on neurologic function is generally an advancing loss of neurologic function and brainstem reflexes. Exceptions exist, and Lloyd (4,5) reported a confused patient with a core temperature of 24°C, emphasizing a potentially poor correlation of the degree of hypothermia with level of consciousness. It has generally been accepted that the diagnosis of brain death cannot reliably be made until the core temperature has reached 32°C.

Hypothermia (usually mild) may occur in a setting of an acute neurologic illness in which the patient is no longer protected against the ambient temperature or in a setting of an endocrine crisis such as hypoglycemic coma or coma from hypothyroidism. It is very important to exclude coingestion of drugs. Opioids, barbiturates, benzodiazepines, phenothiazines, tricyclic antidepressants, and lithium may all cause significant hypothermia when a patient is exposed to a cold environment.

Patients with hypothermia are vasoconstricted, may not shiver when core temperature is below 30°C, and may exhibit a profoundly cold axilla ("cold as marble") (4–7). Tachycardia with conversion to bradycardia will occur at a core temperature

TABLE 6-1. *Clinical features associated with hypothermia*

Body core temperature	Central nervous system	Cardiovascular	Respiratory	Neuromuscular
35–32°C	Apathy; dysarthria; impaired judgment	Tachycardia, then progressive bradycardia; cardiac-cycle prolongation; vasoconstriction	Tachypnea, then progressive bradypnea; bronchorrhea; bronchospasm	Increased muscle tone; shivering; ataxia
32–28°C	Decreased level of consciousness; hallucinations; pupillary dilation	Progressive decrease in pulse and cardiac output; increased cardiac arrhythmias; J waves	Hypoventilation; 50% decrease in carbon dioxide production per 8°C drop in temperature; absence of protective airway reflexes; 50% decrease in oxygen consumption	Hyporeflexia; diminishing shivering; rigidity
<28°C	Coma; absent oculocephalic reflexes; absent corneal reflex; absent bulbar reflexes	Hypotension; bradycardia; reentrant dysrhythmias; decreased ventricular arrhythmia; asystole	Pulmonic congestion and edema; apnea	Amobile; areflexia

Adapted from Danzl DF, Pozos RS. Accidental hypothermia. *N Engl J Med* 1994;331:1756–1760, with permission of the Massachusetts Medical Society.

of 28°C, together with J waves (Osborne waves) (Fig. 6-1), but this configuration may be absent in up to 20% of patients and is not specific for hypothermia (3,4,6,8,9). Pupillary dilatation and sluggish light responses occur at core temperatures between 32°C and 28°C, and other brainstem reflexes disappear below 28°C (Table 6-1).

Management of hypothermia should be characterized by aggressive resuscitation. A recent study from Bern, Switzerland, in 32 young hypothermic (less than 28°C) pa-

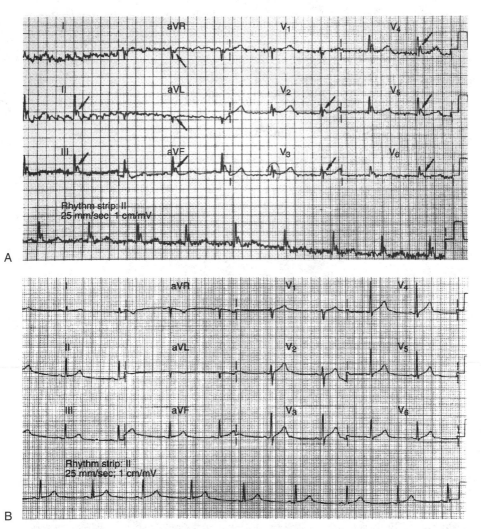

FIG. 6-1. Electrocardiogram showing Osborne waves of hypothermia. **A:** Tracing in a 40-year-old alcoholic with core temperature of 29°C shows bradycardia rhythm (probably sinus), prolonged QT intervals, a baseline artifact due to muscle tremors, and characteristic Osborne waves *(arrows)*. **B:** Sinus rhythm and disappearance of artifact after rewarming to 37.2°C. (From Patel A, Getsos J. Images in clinical medicine. Osborne waves of hypothermia. *N Engl J Med* 1994; 330:680, with permission of the Massachusetts Medical Society.)

tients with circulatory arrest mostly due to mountaineering accidents found no neurologic deficits in 15 resuscitated survivors (7). There is no baseline hypothermia below which resuscitation is invariably unsuccessful. Successful resuscitation with good cognition after 9 h of resuscitative efforts has recently been reported in a patient with a temperature of 13.7°C (10). It is the critical significance of these reports that indicates that an expeditious response is needed, no matter how severe the presenting findings.

Initial management of a mildly hypothermic patient is gentle handling (repeated painful stimuli to assess motor response or grimacing may facilitate the development of cardiac arrhythmias), oxygenation, and crystalloid resuscitation. In most instances, with a core temperature of more than 32°C, rewarming with heating blankets suffices. Extracorporeal rewarming using a cardiopulmonary bypass circuit is indicated when no perfusing cardiac rhythm is present (11,12).

Acute Poisoning

Obviously, toxins, poisons, sedative drugs, and many other agents may cause coma when patients are exposed to large quantities, but only a few pharmaceutical agents have produced a clinical syndrome frighteningly similar to that of structural brain death (13). Barbiturates and tricyclic antidepressants are best known, but in many other instances, certain brainstem reflexes (predominantly pupillary responses) remain intact and make the distinction easy (14–16). Moreover, detailed clinical findings of neurologic examination in intoxicated patients are mostly absent in the literature.

A much more complex problem is the presence of metabolites or traces of circulating pharmaceutical agents, potentially confounding the clinical determination of brain death. Drug screens are helpful, but even though a drug has been identified, a critical threshold is often not known (17–19).

Pupil response to light remains an important distinguishing feature and can be elicited in many cases of poisoning. A magnifying glass may be needed to appreciate pupillary contraction to light. Extreme forms of barbiturate intoxication, however, may result in loss of pupil reaction to light. Mydriasis (8 or 9 mm) or mid-position pupils (6 or 7 mm) can be seen after toxic exposure to antihistamines, tricyclic antidepressants, amphetamines, cocaine, phenylephrine, and other sympathicomimetics. Miosis (1–2 mm) points to any of the anticholinesterase agents, organophosphates, opioids, pilocarpine, and barbiturates. Toxins may induce a structural lesion as a result of anoxia (carbon monoxide), inhibition of phosphorylation (carbon disulfide, cyanide, and hydrogen sulfide), or direct structural neuronal destruction (manganese, 1-methyl-4-phenyl-1,2,3,6-tetrahydropyridine [MPTP]).

Toxins may have a profound and in some instances rather specific effect on other vital organs. Sinus or atrial tachycardia is expected in cocaine, amphetamine, and phencyclidine overdose. Drugs or toxins with anticholinergic effects produce similar tachyarrhythmias (tricyclic antidepressants, scopolomine mushroom and plant ingestion). In the vast majority of patients with tricyclic antidepressant intoxication, there is marked prolongation of the QRS segment of the EKG (15,16).

Pulmonary edema may be falsely attributed to a neurogenic trigger but in fact may be due to the direct effect of toxins. Convincing cases of pulmonary edema exist from heroin, opioids, and many of the hypnotics and sedatives. A cardiodepressant effect is the culprit in most of these instances of pulmonary edema, although a capillary leak syndrome has also been suggested as a potential mechanism (15).

Drug screening and serum quantification of drugs and toxins may assist in assessing their effect on the neurologic examination. Table 6-2 shows the drugs most commonly included in toxicologic screens. Certain toxins are not detectable by emergency toxicologic screens, and important examples are cyanide, lithium, isoniazid, and antibiotics (too polar); aromatic and halogenated hydrocarbon solvents; hydrogen sulfide and nitrogen dioxide (too volatile); and fentanyl, LSD, ergot alkaloids, and digoxin (large volume of distribution and concentration too low) (15,16).

Profound changes in acid–base balance may point to certain kinds of intoxication, and the determination of brain death should be deferred in the presence of acidosis or alkalosis. These derangements may also indicate a possibly reversible medical illness or endocrine crisis. Metabolic acidosis or respiratory acidosis is usually seen in the intoxicated patient and may provide a further helpful guide in identifying the presumed toxin (Table 6-3). The acidosis may be due to uncoupled oxidative phosphorylation (salicylates), seizures (isoniazid, cocaine), or anaerobic glycolysis (cyanide). Pure metabolic or respiratory alkalosis is seldom a manifestation of poisoning.

A reasonable approach can be suggested in drugged patients who actually may be brain dead. First, administer the antidotes naloxone and flumazenil when, respec-

TABLE 6-2. *Drugs included in most toxicologic screens*

Drug type	Examples
Alcohol	Ethanol, methanol, isopropanol, acetone
Barbiturates/sedatives	Amobarbital, secobarbital, pentobarbital, butalbital, butabarbital, phenobarbital, glutethimide, ethchlorvynol, methaqualone
Antiepileptics	Phenytoin, carbamazepine, primadone, phenobarbital
Benzodiazepines	Chlordiazepoxide, diazepam, alprazolam, temazepam
Antihistamines	Diphenhydramine, chlorpheniramine, brompheniramine, tripelennamine, trihexyphenidyl, doxylamine, pyrilamine
Antidepressants	Amitriptyline, nortriptyline, doxepin, imipramine, desipramine, trazodone, amoxapine, maprotiline, fluoxetine
Antipsychotics	Trifluoperazine, perphenazine, prochlorperazine, chlorpromazine
Stimulants	Amphetamine, methamphetamine, phenylpropanolamine, ephedrine, MDA and MDMA (other phenylethylamines), cocaine, phencyclidine
Narcotics, analgesics	Heroin, morphine, codeine, oxycodone, hydrocodone, hydromorphone, meperidine, pentazocine, propoxyphene
Other analgesics	Salicylates, acetaminophen
Cardiovascular drugs	Lidocaine, propranolol, metoprolol, quinidine, procainamide, verapamil
Others	Theophylline, caffeine, nicotine, oral hypoglycemics, strychnine

TABLE 6-3. *Drug-induced acid-base abnormalities*

Metabolic acidosis
    Acetaminophen
    Ethanol, methanol, ethylene glycol
    Salicylates
    Isoniazid
    Cyanide
    Cocaine
    Strychnine
    Papaverine
    Toluene
Respiratory acidosis
    Opiates
    Ethanol, other alcohols
    Barbiturates
    Anesthetics

tively, opioids or benzodiazepines have been administered and look for change. In cases highly suspicious for carbon monoxide intoxication, administer oxygen; for intoxication due to carbon disulfide, cyanide, and hydrogen sulfide, use amyl nitrite. Second, declare brain death if a screening test reveals traces of a drug below the therapeutic range. (Thus, for example, one should accept as noncontributory the presence of antiepileptic agents in levels below therapeutic range and alcohol in levels below the legal limit of drunken driving.) Third, when the drug or poison cannot be quantified but is certain, observe the patient for at least four times the excretion half-life, provided elimination of the drug or toxin is not interfered with by other drugs or organ dysfunction (e.g., cocaine, 4 h; thiopental, 40 h) (Table 6-4). When the drug is not known but suspicion of its presence remains high, observe the patient for 48 h for a change in brainstem reflexes and motor response; if none are observed, perform a confirmatory test for brain death (preferably documenting absence of intracranial flow with a cerebral angiogram).

The most common clinical dilemma is the diagnosis of brain death in a patient with traumatic brain injury with no brainstem function, a computed tomography (CT) scan showing massive brain destruction and documented serum pentobarbital levels. Replacing clinical examination with a cerebral angiogram is ill advised. When high-dose barbiturates are used, depressed neuronal function and decreased cerebral blood flow (due to its coupling) may occur. Significant reduction in cerebral blood flow theoretically may impair contrast filling, though the evidence is equivocal. The clinical diagnosis of brain death should only be allowed if serum pentobarbital levels have decreased to levels in which it is highly improbable that brainstem function is depressed (usually, in most laboratories, less than 5 μg/mL).

Acute Metabolic Encephalopathies

As in poisoning, neurologic accounts of acute metabolic encephalopathy mimicking brain death are sketchy and devoid of details. Acute metabolic derangements,

TABLE 6-4. *Drugs that may confound neurologic examination in brain death*

Drugs	Plasma $t^{1/2}$ (h)	Therapeutic range
Lorazepam	10–20	0.1–0.3 µg/mL
Clonazepam	20–30	10–50 ng/mL
Midazolam	2–5	50–150 ng/mL
Flurazepam	70–100	100–500 ng/mL
Diazepam	40	0.2–0.8 µg/mL
Phenytoin	≥140	10–20 µg/mL
Chlordiazepoxide	10–12	1–3 µg/mL
Carbamazepine	10–60	2–10 µg/mL
Valproic acid	15–20	40–100 µg/mL
Phenobarbital	100	20–40 µg/mL
Thiopental	10	6–35 µg/mL
Pentobarbital	10	1–5 µg/mL
Primidone	15–20	9–12 µg/mL
Morphine	2–3	70–450 ng/mL
Fentanyl	18–60	NA
Ketamine	2–4	NA
Amitriptyline	10–24	75–200 ng/mL
Pancuronium[a]	2–3	NA
Vecuronium[a]	2–3	NA
Pipecuronium[a]	2–3	NA
Alcohol[b]	10 mL/h	800–1,500 mg/L
Cocaine	1	150–300 ng/mL
Codeine	3	200–350 ng/mL

[a] Peripheral nerve stimulation may be helpful. When all twitches in a train of four stimuli are present, it is unlikely that neuromuscular junction blockers are major confounders.

[b] Plasma $t^{1/2}$ may easily change as a result of interacting drugs and organ failure. Use legal alcohol limit for determination of brain death.

NA, not available.

endocrine crises, or other acute organ failure may result in a clinical diagnosis of brain death, mostly only after structural damage. Typically, diffuse cerebral edema, extensive demyelination, or anoxic-ischemic injury may result in an irreversible brain injury and subsequently progress to brain death (20,21). Examples are brain edema in fulminant hepatic failure and ketotic hyperglycemia and the emergence of pontine and extrapontine demyelination due to treatment of severe hyponatremia. However, severe hyponatremia, hypernatremia, hyperglycemia or hypoglycemia, hypothyroidism, panhypopituitarism, or adrenal dysfunction could result in a profound decrease in the level of consciousness, seizures, or status epilepticus and occasionally localizing signs but not complete loss of brainstem reflexes. Patients who fulfill the criteria of brain death may have some degree of hypernatremia from diabetes insipidus and hyperglycemia due to the sympathetic stress response induced by brain destruction, but these abnormalities, if not severe, should be considered secondary.

Isolated Medulla Oblongata

Traditionally, deterioration in brain herniation follows a pattern in which the mesencephalon, pons, and medulla oblongata subsequently cease to function, although loss of all medulla function may take hours to complete. In exceptional cases, the progression of herniation may halt at the level of the medulla oblongata.

Retained medulla oblongata function can be suspected in a patient who has lost most brainstem reflexes but whose blood pressure is unsupported and who has occasional cough responses. Breathing is intact after disconnection from the ventilator, and cough reflexes with deep tracheobronchial suctioning are present. When 1 mg of atropine is administered, tachycardia may be observed (22).

A few cases have been published of spontaneous breathing during the apnea test in patients who have fulfilled all other clinical criteria of brain death. Notably, Ropper et al. (23) reported four cases with sparing of only the medulla oblongata as indicated by normal respirations, and these patients survived for several days to 3 weeks with stable unsupported blood pressures.

This condition of partial retained function of the medulla oblongata ("medulla man") precludes a diagnosis of brain death (24).

Illustrative Case Report

Following a motor vehicle accident and submersion in water, the Glasgow coma sum score of this patient was 3 on arrival at the hospital, the left pupil was dilated with a diameter of 8 mm, fixed to light, and oculocephalic reflexes were absent (24). CT scan showed a large left epidural supratentorial hematoma with a shift of midline structures and effaced basal cisterns.

After evacuation of an epidural hematoma, the patient remained comatose. Repeat CT scan showed a new stellate hematoma in the pons (Fig. 6-2). Brainstem reflexes were absent except for a major discrepancy in eliciting the cough response. Up and down movements of an endotracheal tube were negative, but suctioning with introduction of a tube to the carina or main bronchus level produced a cough response. An apnea test was performed after disconnection from the ventilator and with appropriate precautions and preoxygenation. A spontaneous regular respiratory effort with tidal volumes between 300 and 500 mL was noted at a $Paco_2$ of 34 mm Hg, and the test was terminated. This clinical condition persisted for the next 48 h. Two additional apnea tests at 12-h intervals produced similar results. The family decided to withdraw support, and the patient was placed on a T-piece with 4 L of oxygen. For an additional 8 h, the patient had normal respiratory drive but was intermittently tachypneic with respiratory rates varying from 20 to 30 per minute. Oxygenation measured by pulse oximetry remained normal. Blood pressures stabilized at 90 to 100 mm Hg systolic without pharmacologic support.

The family decided to have the patient extubated, which resulted in respiratory arrest. Pathologic examination revealed multiple shear lesions and a primary traumatic pontine lesion but no macroscopic or microscopic medulla oblongata lesion (Fig. 6-2), although tonsillar herniation had resulted in some compression of the medulla oblongata.

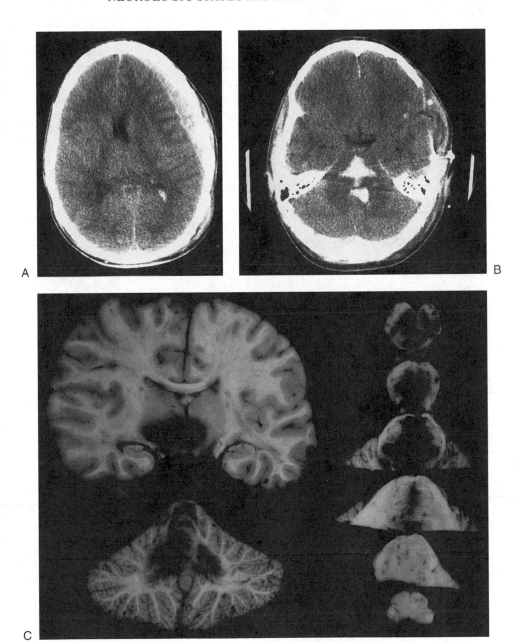

FIG. 6-2. Computed tomography scans show left frontal epidural hematoma **(A)** and stellate pontine hemorrhage and intraventricular hemorrhage **(B). C:** Pathologic confirmation of normal medulla oblongata despite multiple brain and brainstem and cerebellar lesions. (From Wijdicks EFM, Atkinson JLD, Okazaki H, et al. Isolated medulla oblongata function after severe traumatic brain injury. *J Neurol Neurosurg Psychiatry* 2001;70:127–129, with permission of the publisher.)

The presence of this comatose state so closely resembling brain death reinforces the need not only for apnea testing but also for careful evaluation of cough reflexes and other medullary function. Failure to examine cough responses with bronchial suctioning or deferral of a formal apnea test may lead to an incorrect clinical diagnosis of brain death. The presence of an intact or only partly damaged medulla oblongata may provide some regulation of cardiovascular, respiratory, and autonomic function and may "stabilize" the patient's condition. Progressive loss of hemodynamic systems and finally cardiac arrest, as expected in brain death, may not occur.

RELATED NEUROLOGIC DISORDERS

This section discusses disorders that contrast with brain death. They are included here to explore the various kinds of impact that destructive lesions may have on brain function, but a slipup in diagnosis is not defensible.

Akinetic Mutism

In this rather unusual comatose state, there is pathologically slowed or nearly absent bodily movement and loss of speech but with some rudimentary wakefulness and self-awareness (20,25). Sleep and wake cycles are intact. There is experience of suffering. Respiratory function is normal. Patients with akinetic mutism may register speech and exceptionally may answer with "yes" and "no." The condition has been given the connotation "motionless, mindless, wakefulness" by Cairns and associates (26) in the original description in 1941. In that report, a young female patient with a cyst in the third ventricle became mute and did not move but reacted adequately to external stimuli; she recovered after ventricular shunting. More recently, a similar case with improvement after shunting was reported by Abekura (27), who described a 12-year-old boy with obstructive hydrocephalus who became mute, bradykinetic, and immobile, fell asleep easily, exhibited a blank stare, and had significant vertical eye movement abnormalities. An MRI scan showed obstructive hydrocephalus due to malfunction of the ventriculoperitoneal shunt.

Akinetic mutism is anatomically divided into frontal and mesencephalic types. The frontal type is most typically seen in patients with infarction in the distribution of the anterior communicating cerebral artery. Associated conditions are aneurysmal subarachnoid hemorrhage, multiple cerebral infarcts from atrial fibrillation, episodes of severe hypotension, or hypercoagulable states (28–31). Cerebral infarction may involve not only the basomedial frontal lobe but also the orbital cortex, the septal area, and particularly the cingulate gyri. Bithalamic infarction has also been documented in patients with akinetic mutism. The central part of the thalamus is most severely affected, including the intralaminar and midline nuclei, whose fibers diverge to the region of the cortex and involve motor execution. The mesencephalic type of akinetic mutism additionally shows vertical gaze palsy and ophthalmoplegia, and these features clinically distinguish this type from the more traditional frontal lesion.

More recently, potentially reversible toxic causes of akinetic mutism have been described and included baclofen and cyclosporin A (32–35). Amphotericin-B–associated leukoencephalopathy was seen in patients with akinetic mutism who underwent bone marrow transplantation, with autopsy findings showing widespread myelin loss in the centrum semiovale, operculum, white matter, and external capsules. Cyclosporin A neurotoxicity may result in severe pseudobulbar palsy that progresses to akinetic mutism, with complete recovery after withdrawal of the drug and, surprisingly, no recurrence after its reintroduction (36,37). Akinetic mutism has also been described in the setting of necrotizing leukoencephalopathy after irradiation and chemotherapy.

Some improvement is possible, and patients with akinetic mutism can evolve into a severely disabled state with effective communication. In a recent case report (38), bromocriptine and ephedrine were used to compensate for damage to the ascending monoamine projections. A gradual increase of dosage of bromocriptine to 27.5 mg orally every 6 h and of ephedrine 25 mg three times daily resulted in significant improvement in communication and recall. Total maintainance was bromocriptine 100 mg/day and ephedrine 525 mg/day. Experience with these drugs remains anecdotal.

Persistent Vegetative State

It may seem contrary to all reasonable expectation that patients in a persistent vegetative state with intact brainstem function, breathing drive, and blood pressure regulation can be judged to be brain dead. This misunderstanding may have its origin in the interchangeable lay use of the terms "brain dead" and "vegetable." Jennett and Plum coined the term "persistent vegetative state" and eloquently delineated its salient features. Plum recently explained that the term "vegetative" was taken from Bichat's earlier work on the nervous system, long before the autonomic nervous system was recognized, in which Bichat separated a vegetative component, indicating thereby the neurovascular and nutritional system (39).

The notion of a vegetative state has recently been scrutinized by a multisociety task force (40). The resulting landmark document assimilates available scientific data on presentation and on diagnosis and outcome. Its real contribution, however, is the way it expanded the definition and introduced a new term in the medical lexicon: "permanent vegetative state" (irreversible) as distinguished from "persistent vegetative state" (yet uncertain outcome). The persistent vegetative state is defined as "a clinical condition of complete unawareness of the self and environment accompanied by sleep-wake cycles with either complete or partial preservation of the hypothalamic and brain-stem autonomic functions" (Table 6-5). Any acute catastrophic brain injury can result in a persistent vegetative state, but the condition is rare, contrary to public perception. Traumatic brain injuries, including gunshot wounds, are the most frequent causative injuries. Nontraumatic injuries are usually due to hypoxic-ischemic injury resulting from cardiorespiratory arrest, asphyxia or near drowning, subarachnoid hemorrhage, meningitis, or encephalitis and, less commonly, from toxins or poisons in the central nervous system. Many degenerative disorders and inborn errors may eventually lead to a persistent vegetative state.

TABLE 6-5. *Clinical criteria for the persistent-permanent vegetative state*

Time duration: 1 month; if persistent more than 1 year, almost always permanent
Function lost:
  No cognition: consistent responses to linguistic, symbolic, or mimetic instruction are absent
  No semantically meaningful sounds or goal-directed movements
  No sustained head-ocular pursuit activity
Functions usually or often preserved:
  Brainstem and autonomically controlled visceral functions: homeothermia; osmolar homeo-
    stasis; breathing; circulation; gastrointestinal functions
  Pupillary and oculovestibular reflexes usually remain and are accentuated
  Brief, inconsistent shifting of head or eyes toward new sounds or sights may occur
  Smiles, tears, or rage reactions may occur either spontaneously or to nonverbal sounds
  Reflex postural responses to noxious stimuli remain

From Plum F, Schiff N, Ribar U, et al. Coordinated expression in chronically unconscious persons. *Phil Trans R Soc Lond B Biol Sci* 1998;353:1929–1933, with permission of the Royal Society.

Patients in a vegetative state have their eyes open ("wakefulness without awareness"); have preserved brainstem reflexes as well as breathing; show no evidence of
sustained, reproducible, purposeful, or voluntary behavioral response to visual, auditory, tactile, or noxious stimuli; show no evidence of language comprehension or expression; have bowel and bladder incontinence; and have variable preserved cranial
nerve and spinal reflexes (Table 6-5) (40). Neurologic examination in a patient in a
vegetative state is predicated on the absence of awareness, but random movements of
the extremities may be seen, along with grimacing and smiling, grunting, moaning
and screaming, and startle myoclonus. The vegetative state is distinguished from
other comatose conditions by a lack of any sustained visual pursuit (41,42). There is
no fixation on a visual target or tracking of objects. Gagging, coughing, sucking, and
swallowing reflexes are preserved but are insufficient, and these patients require tube
feeding to prevent aspiration. Some patients may continue to randomly utter single
words or have stereotypical, purposeless, coordinated chorea-like movements or rage
reactions with high-pitched screaming, clenching of teeth when stimulated, flushing
of skin, and increase in blood pressure. Some patients may inconsistently turn their
head toward a loud sound, but positron emission tomography (PET) studies have
documented failure to activate auditory processing in the cortex (43). Persistent vegetative state may be delineated from a "minimally conscious state," in which, though
the disability is very severe, some object-directed feedback exists (41).

Neuroimaging and cerebral blood flow studies in patients in a persistent vegetative
state have confirmed the presence of profound brain damage. Recent magnetic resonance imaging (MRI) studies in patients with persistent vegetative state after closed
head injury demonstrated not only profound scattered hemispheric lesions but also
frequent corpus callosum and primary dorsolateral brainstem lesions (44).

PET studies showed glucose metabolic rates 30% to 50% lower than controls, but
these "anesthesia-like" metabolic rates may not greatly correlate with neurologic
functioning, which can only be assessed clinically and over time (39,45). Further insight into the extent of neuronal loss and changes in thalamocortical connections dur-

ing recovery from persistent vegetative states has come from two recent PET studies and when confirmed may have an important role in prediction. One study of an "acute vegetative state" due to an anoxic-ischemic insult (defined as a vegetative state less than 1 month in duration) found that recovery was highly unlikely when cortical flumazenil binding to cortical benzodiazepine receptors was five times below average values. In this study, neuronal integrity was evaluated by using ^{11}C-flumazenil and assessing the density of cortical benzodiazepine receptors (46). A second study, using $H_2^{15}O$ PET studies, showed resumption of the functional relation between thalamic and associative cortex in patients who recovered consciousness (47). Diffuse laminar cortical necrosis (Fig. 6-3) and traumatic diffuse axonal injury can be expected in the majority of patients when they come to autopsy months to years after the initial insult.

Neuropathologic studies in persistent-permanent vegetative state are determined by the underlying destructive lesion. Kinney and Samuels (48) suggested that the cortex is "locked-out" and disconnected as a result of damage to the cerebral cortex, subcortical connections from either axonal or myelin injury of the white matter, and thalamus.

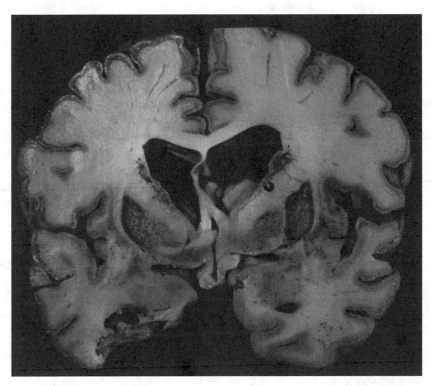

FIG. 6-3. Pathologic specimen of a patient who survived in a vegetative state but for a short time. The cerebral cortex is thin, and neuronal loss producing cavities in the putamen is seen in conjunction with enlarged *(ex vacuo)* ventricles.

Disproportionate involvement of the thalamus has been reported with largely intact basal forebrain, brainstem, and hypothalamus. This observation from the carefully documented autopsy of Karen Ann Quinlan corroborates the current hypothesis that the thalamic reticular nucleus plays a pivotal role in arousal (49). In addition, a recent neuropathology study from the Institute of Neurological Sciences in Glasgow found thalamic lesions in 80% and ischemic lesions in multiple neocortical territories in 43% of patients in a vegetative state (50,51). Both ischemic (neuronal loss in anterior and dorsomedial nuclei) and traumatic (neuronal loss in lateral and ventral nuclei) thalamus lesions were found (50).

The confrontation of families with such a state is immeasurably painful. It may be thought of as a funeral on hold. However, the mortality from persistent vegetative state in adults is very high, and prolonged survival is uncommon (mortality, 82% at 3 years and 95% at 5 years). On the other hand, "improvement" to a severely disabled state in traumatic head injury after 3 months is still more than 50%. In contrast, nontraumatic insults to the brain resulting in persistent vegetative state for at least 3 months have a much worse prospect, with only 7% recovery to a severely disabled state at 3 months and, very rarely, reported cases of recovery after 6 months (40). From time to time, "improvement" to a moderately or severely disabled state after 12 months has been described, but only in a few younger patients, mainly less than 45 years of age.

Locked-In Syndrome

Locked-in syndrome is a consequence of destruction of the base of the pons. Consciousness is intact, but the patient is unable to move his or her extremities, grimace, or swallow, but is able to blink and move eyes vertically. There is no intellectual decline, and surviving patients can function with devices. Often, blinking is noted, either spontaneously with touching of eyelashes, after a loud sound, or by serendipity. Vertical eye movements become apparent when the patient is asked to look up or down. Quickening of the heart rate after noxious pain stimulus, typically absent in brain death, should point to a different condition as well. The most common diagnostic errors are made in patients who have hemorrhage in the pons or cerebellum, embolus to the basilar artery, or any tumors that compress the brainstem.

The term "locked-in syndrome" was introduced by Plum and Posner in 1966 to replace other terms, such as pontopseudocoma, ventral pontine syndrome, de-efferented state, pontine disconnection syndrome, and Montecristo syndrome (referring to Monsieur Noirtier, who was in this state for more than 6 years and was described as a "corpse with living eyes") (20). Earlier descriptions of a locked-in syndrome include that by Emile Zola in his novel Thérèse Raquin, in which Madame Raquin had a stroke. The features of the syndrome are nicely summarized by Pearce as "her tongue turned to stone," "she was struck dumb and motionless," "she only had the language of her eyes," and "she could communicate quite easily with an imprisoned mind buried alive in a dead body" (52). The most recent dramatic and sad description of locked-in syndrome is that by Jean-Dominique Bauby, editor-in-chief of the Parisian magazine *Elle*, who had a devastating stroke in the brainstem. His book is titled *The Diving Bell and the Butterfly,* referring to the heavy corporeal trap—the "Diving Bell"—and his imagination wandering off in space or time—the lightness of a "Butterfly." Bauby often strove to savor the pleasures that were left to him, such as smells and vision. With a feat of great will power, he blinked more than 200,000 times to produce a 137-page book describing his ordeal before he died (53). The book provides useful insight into the cruelty and terror of this condition.

The pathologic lesion in locked-in syndrome interrupts the corticobulbar and corticospinal tracts, but the tegmentum of the pons and mid brain, which harbors the reticular formation, is preserved, and thus consciousness is fully retained (54–56). Voluntary eye movements in the vertical plane and blinking remain because the oculomotor and trochlear nuclei and the center for vertical gaze remain intact. A significant skew deviation may occur along with ocular bobbing, both of which may be additional visual handicaps. Even further limitation of communication has been reported by Keane (57), who encountered a patient with a pontine hemorrhage who had locked-in syndrome and was also deaf. In others, remnants of pontine function may be present. In these patients, bilateral extensor posturing and horizontal ocular eye movements, sometimes with only a trace of abduction, are present.

In patients with a basilar artery occlusion, extension of the infarct into the tegmentum and involvement of the thalamus may further decrease the level of consciousness. The characteristic alertness in locked-in syndrome may also be significantly confounded by sedative agents used for mechanical ventilation. Locked-in syndrome may not be recognized in patients who appear motionless.

The causes of locked-in syndrome are summarized in Table 6-6 (55,57–70). Basilar artery occlusion is a common etiology, which in young patients is largely due to vertebral artery dissection. One may distinguish a central from a peripheral form of locked-in syndrome. Obviously, in the peripheral type, vertical eye movements and blinking are additionally absent. Most vivid examples are patients with a rapidly progressive Guillain-Barré syndrome and patients who have received neuromuscular-blocking agents during general anesthesia but cannot eliminate them because of a defect in metabolism.

TABLE 6-6. *Causes of "locked-in syndrome"*

Central
    Basilar artery occlusion
    Fulminant demyelinating disease
    Glioma
    Uncal herniation
    Head injury
    Pontine abscess
    Pontine hemorrhage
    Herpes (brainstem) encephalitis
    Central pontine myelinolysis
Peripheral
    Guillain-Barré syndrome
    Organophosphate poisoning
    Neuromuscular-blocking agents
    Advanced amyotrophic lateral sclerosis

MRI is the preferred imaging modality in locked-in syndrome (Fig. 6-4). It may show involvement of the base of the pons, extention into the mesencephalon, and sparing of the tegmentum. Electroencephalographic (EEG) reactivity in locked-in syndrome is most often preserved (71). Recently, Gütling et al. (66) reported absent EEG reactivity in some cases, but these patients also had damage to cortical structures, and it is possible that absent EEG reactivity may indicate extension to the pontine tegmentum. One preliminary study (71) also showed that preservation of motor-evoked potentials in the acute phase may herald a good recovery, but the technique is not widely available (71). In a study of sleep patterns in locked-in syndrome us-

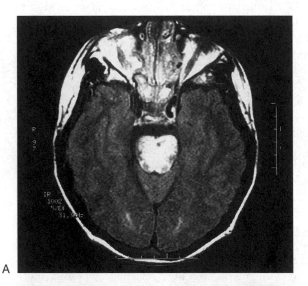

A

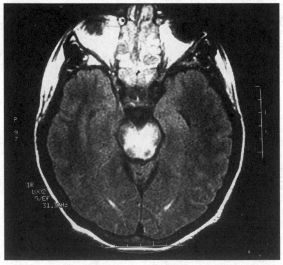

B

FIG. 6-4. Patient with locked in syndrome. Fluid-attenuated inversion recovery sequence magnetic resonance imaging: T$_2$ signal abnormality within brainstem pons **(A)** and mesencephalon **(B)**, with sparing of tegmentum **(C)**. *(continued)*

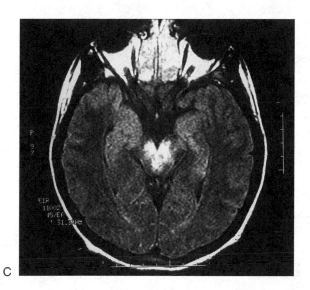

C

FIG. 6-4. *Continued.*

ing polysomnography, only minor abnormalities were noted, which raises the interesting question whether the upper half of the pons plays a role in sleep regulation (72).

A large proportion of patients die from pulmonary complications, but some patients have survived for many years, including one for up to 27 years (59,73). This particular case is of interest because the patient survived major medical complications, including intestinal obstruction, gram-negative sepsis, upper gastrointestinal bleeding, septic arthritis, and recurrent urinary tract infections. In most patients, the locked-in state remains unchanged. Some improvement may occur, such as movement of fingers which allows better signaling. Spasm of the jaw musculature has been noted, as have postures that are fragments of the extensor spasms of cerebrate rigidity. However, recovery from locked-in syndrome has been reported in patients with herpes simplex encephalitis (74), after a bout of basilar artery migraine (75,76), and following uncal herniation from a lobar hematoma (77). In most of these cases, improvement occurred within days to weeks after presentation. Late recovery has not been reported (78).

CONCLUSION

Several medical conditions may superficially mimic brain death from structural destructive lesion. Except for hypothermia and, rarely, drug intoxication, careful neurologic examination should quickly reveal a different comatose state. In most of these disorders, breathing drive remains normal.

REFERENCES

1. Van Norman GA. A matter of life and death: what every anesthesiologist should know about the medical, legal, and ethical aspects of declaring brain death. *Anesthesiology* 1999;91:275–287.

2. Youngner SJ, Landefeld CS, Coulton CJ, et al. "Brain death" and organ retrieval. A cross-sectional survey of knowledge and concepts among health professionals. *JAMA* 1989;261:2205–2210.
3. Weinberg AD. Hypothermia. *Ann Emerg Med* 1993;22:370–377.
4. Lloyd EL. Accidental hypothermia. *Resuscitation* 1996;32:111–124.
5. Lloyd EL. Accidental hypothermia treated by central rewarming through the airway. *Br J Anaesth* 1973;45:41–48.
6. Patel A, Getsos J. Images in clinical medicine. Osborn waves of hypothermia. *N Engl J Med* 1994; 330:680.
7. Walpoth BH, Walpoth-Aslan BN, Mattle HP, et al. Outcome of survivors of accidental deep hypothermia and circulatory arrest treated with extracorporeal blood warming. *N Engl J Med* 1997; 337:1500–1505.
8. Danzl DF, Pozos RS. Accidental hypothermia. *N Engl J Med* 1994;331:1756–1760.
9. Patel A, Getsos JP, Moussa G, et al. The Osborn wave of hypothermia in normothermic patients. *Clin Cardiol* 1994;17:273–276.
10. Gilbert M, Busund R, Skagseth A, et al. Resuscitation from accidental hypothermia of 13.7 degrees C with circulatory arrest [Letter]. *Lancet* 2000;355:375–376.
11. Larach MG. Accidental hypothermia. *Lancet* 1995;345:493–498.
12. Deakin CD. Forced air surface rewarming in patients with severe accidental hypothermia [Letter]. *Resuscitation* 2000;43:223.
13. Morris RG. Drugs and brain death: drug assay perspectives. *Clin Exp Pharmacol Physiol* 1996; 23:S42–S43.
14. Yang KL, Dantzker DR. Reversible brain death. A manifestation of amitriptyline overdose. *Chest* 1991;99:1037–1038.
15. Ellenhorn MJ, Barceloux DG, Schonwald S, et al, eds. *Ellenhorn's medical toxicology: diagnosis and treatment of human poisoning,* 2nd ed. Baltimore: Williams & Wilkins, 1997.
16. Goldfrank LR, Flomenbaum NE, Lewin NA, et al, eds. *Goldfrank's toxicologic emergencies,* 6th ed. Stamford, CT: Appleton & Lange, 1998.
17. Flanagan RJ. The poisoned patient: the role of the laboratory. *Br J Biomed Sci* 1995;52:202–213.
18. Watson ID. Laboratory support for the poisoned patient. *Ther Drug Monit* 1998;20:490–497.
19. Volans G, Widdop B. ABC of poisoning. Laboratory investigations in acute poisoning. *BMJ* 1984; 289:426–428.
20. Plum F, Posner JB, eds. *The diagnosis of stupor and coma,* 3rd ed. Philadelphia: FA Davis Company, 1980.
21. Wijdicks EFM. *Neurology of critical illness.* Philadelphia: FA Davis Company, 1995.
22. Ouaknine GE. Bedside procedures in the diagnosis of brain death. *Resuscitation* 1975;4:159–177.
23. Ropper AH, Kennedy SK, Russell L. Apnea testing in the diagnosis of brain death. Clinical and physiological observations. *J Neurosurg* 1981;55:942–946.
24. Wijdicks EFM, Atkinson JLD, Okazaki H. Isolated medulla oblongata after severe traumatic brain injury. *J Neurol Neurosurg Psychiatry* 2001;70:127–129.
25. Ure J, Faccio E, Videla H, et al. Akinetic mutism: a report of three cases. *Acta Neurol Scand* 1998; 98:439–444.
26. Cairns H, Oldfield RC, Pennybacker JB, et al. Akinetic mutism with epidermoid cyst of third ventricle (with report on associated disturbance of brain potentials). *Brain* 1941;64:273–290.
27. Abekura M. Akinetic mutism and magnetic resonance imaging in obstructive hydrocephalus. Case illustration. *J Neurosurg* 1998;88:161.
28. van Domburg PH, ten Donkelaar HJ, Notermans SL. Akinetic mutism with bithalamic infarction. Neurophysiological correlates. *J Neurol Sci* 1996;139:58–65.
29. Fesenmeier JT, Kuzniecky R, Garcia JH. Akinetic mutism caused by bilateral anterior cerebral tuberculous obliterative arteritis. *Neurology* 1990;40:1005–1006.
30. Minagar A, David NJ. Bilateral infarction in the territory of the anterior cerebral arteries. *Neurology* 1999;52:886–888.
31. Nagaratnam N, McNeil C, Gilhotra JS. Akinetic mutism and mixed transcortical aphasia following left thalamo-mesencephalic infarction. *J Neurol Sci* 1999;163:70–73.
32. Devinsky O, Lemann W, Evans AC, et al. Akinetic mutism in a bone marrow transplant recipient following total-body irradiation and amphotericin B chemoprophylaxis. A positron emission tomographic and neuropathologic study. *Arch Neurol* 1987;44:414–417.
33. Rubin DI, So EL. Reversible akinetic mutism possibly induced by baclofen. *Pharmacotherapy* 1999; 19:468–470.
34. Walker RW, Rosenblum MK. Amphotericin B–associated leukoencephalopathy. *Neurology* 1992; 42:2005–2010.

35. Parmar MS. Akinetic mutism after baclofen [Letter]. *Ann Intern Med* 1991;115:499–500.
36. Bronster DJ, Boccagni P, O'Rourke M, et al. Loss of speech after orthotopic liver transplantation. *Transplant Int* 1995;8:234–237.
37. Bird GL, Meadows J, Goka J, et al. Cyclosporin-associated akinetic mutism and extrapyramidal syndrome after liver transplantation. *J Neurol Neurosurg Psychiatry* 1990;53:1068–1071.
38. Anderson B. Relief of akinetic mutism from obstructive hydrocephalus using bromocriptine and ephedrine. Case report. *J Neurosurg* 1992;76:152–155.
39. Plum F, Schiff N, Ribary U, et al. Coordinated expression in chronically unconscious persons. *Philos Trans R Soc Lond B Biol Sci* 1998;353:1929–1933.
40. The Multi-Society Task Force on PVS. Medical aspects of the persistent vegetative state (parts 1 and 2). *N Engl J Med* 1994;330:1499–1508,1572–1579.
41. Giacino JT. Disorders of consciousness: differential diagnosis and neuropathologic features. *Semin Neurol* 1997;17:105–111.
42. Tommasino C. Coma and vegetative state are not interchangeable terms [Letter]. *Anesthesiology* 1995;83:888–889.
43. Laureys S, Faymonville M-E, Degueldre C, et al. Auditory processing in the vegetative state. *Brain* 2000;123:1589–1601.
44. Kampfl A, Schmutzhard E, Franz G, et al. Prediction of recovery from post-traumatic vegetative state with cerebral magnetic-resonance imaging. *Lancet* 1998;351:1763–1767.
45. Levy DE, Sidtis JJ, Rottenberg DA, et al. Differences in cerebral blood flow and glucose utilization in vegetative versus locked-in patients. *Ann Neurol* 1987;22:673–682.
46. Rudolf J, Sobesky J, Grond M, et al. Identification by positron emission tomography of neuronal loss in acute vegetative state [Letter]. *Lancet* 2000;355:115–116.
47. Laureys S, Faymonville ME, Luxen A, et al. Restoration of thalamocortical connectivity after recovery from persistent vegetative state [Letter]. *Lancet* 2000;355:1790–1791.
48. Kinney HC, Samuels MA. Neuropathology of the persistent vegetative state. A review. *J Neuropathol Exp Neurol* 1994;53:548–558.
49. Kinney HC, Korein J, Panigrahy A, et al. Neuropathological findings in the brain of Karen Ann Quinlan. The role of the thalamus in the persistent vegetative state. *N Engl J Med* 1994;330:1469–1475.
50. Adams JH, Jennett B, McLellan DR, et al. The neuropathology of the vegetative state after head injury. *J Clin Pathol* 1999;52:804–806.
51. Adams JH, Graham DI, Jennett B. The neuropathology of the vegetative state after an acute brain insult. *Brain* 2000;123:1327–1338.
52. Pearce JM. The locked in syndrome [Editorial]. *BMJ* 1987;294:198–199.
53. Bauby J-D, ed. *The diving bell and the butterfly.* (French translation by Jeremy Leggatt.) New York: Knopf, 1997.
54. Ohry A. The locked-in syndrome and related states [Editorial]. *Paraplegia* 1990;28:73–75.
55. Patterson JR, Grabois M. Locked-in syndrome: a review of 139 cases. *Stroke* 1986;17:758–764.
56. Reznik M. Neuropathology in seven cases of locked-in syndrome. *J Neurol Sci* 1983;60:67–78.
57. Keane JR. Locked-in syndrome with deafness [Letter]. *Neurology* 1985;35:1395.
58. Chia LG. Locked-in syndrome with bilateral ventral midbrain infarcts. *Neurology* 1991;41:445–446.
59. Dollfus P, Milos PL, Chapuis A, et al. The locked-in syndrome: a review and presentation of two chronic cases. *Paraplegia* 1990;28:5–16.
60. Keane JR, Itabashi HH. Locked-in syndrome due to tentorial herniation. *Neurology* 1985;35:1647–1649.
61. Larmande P, Henin D, Jan M, et al. Abnormal vertical eye movements in the locked-in syndrome. *Ann Neurol* 1982;11:100–102.
62. Marti-Masso JF, Suarez J, Lopez de Munain A, et al. Clinical signs of brain death simulated by Guillain-Barré syndrome. *J Neurol Sci* 1993;120:115–117.
63. Tijssen CC, Ter Bruggen JP. Locked-in syndrome associated with ocular bobbing. *Acta Neurol Scand* 1986;73:444–446.
64. Feldman MH. Physiological observations in a chronic case of "locked-in" syndrome. *Neurology* 1971;21:459–478.
65. Haig AJ, Katz RT, Sahgal V. Mortality and complications of the locked-in syndrome. *Arch Phys Med Rehabil* 1987;68:24–27.
66. Gütling E, Isenmann S, Wichmann W. Electrophysiology in the locked-in syndrome. *Neurology* 1996;46:1092–1101.
67. Bakshi N, Maselli RA, Gospe SM Jr, et al. Fulminant demyelinating neuropathy mimicking cerebral death. *Muscle Nerve* 1997;20:1595–1597.

68. Bivins D, Biller J, Laster DW, et al. Recovery from posttraumatic locked-in syndrome with basilar artery occlusion. *Surg Neurol* 1981;16:230–234.
69. Blunt SB, Boulton J, Wise R, et al. Locked-in syndrome in fulminant demyelinating disease [Letter]. *J Neurol Neurosurg Psychiatry* 1994;57:504–505.
70. Forti A, Ambrosetto G, Amore M, et al. Locked-in syndrome in multiple sclerosis with sparing of the ventral portion of the pons. *Ann Neurol* 1982;12:393–394.
71. Bassetti C, Mathis J, Hess CW. Multimodal electrophysiological studies including motor evoked potentials in patients with locked-in syndrome: report of six patients. *J Neurol Neurosurg Psychiatry* 1994;57:1403–1406.
72. Oksenberg A, Soroker N, Solzi P, et al. Polysomnography in locked-in syndrome. *Electroencephalogr Clin Neurophysiol* 1991;78:314–317.
73. Thadani VM, Rimm DL, Urquhart L, et al. "Locked-in syndrome" for 27 years following a viral illness: clinical and pathologic findings. *Neurology* 1991;41:498–500.
74. Matsumura K, Sakuta M. Oculogyric crisis in acute herpetic brainstem encephalitis [Letter]. *J Neurol Neurosurg Psychiatry* 1987;50:365–366.
75. Buchman AS, Wichter MD. Recovery following the "locked-in" syndrome [Letter]. *Stroke* 1986; 17:558.
76. Sulkava R, Kovanen J. Locked-in syndrome with rapid recovery: a manifestation of basilar artery migraine? *Headache* 1983;23:238–239.
77. Wijdicks EFM, Miller GM. Transient locked-in syndrome after uncal herniation. *Neurology* 1999; 52:1296–1297.
78. Cappa SF, Vignolo LA. Locked-in syndrome for 12 years with preserved intelligence [Letter]. *Ann Neurol* 1982;11:545.

7

Religious and Cultural Aspects of Brain Death

Christine M. Gallagher[*] and Eelco F. M. Wijdicks[†]

*Religious Outreach Consultant, Grand Junction, Colorado, and †Department of Neurology, Mayo Clinic, Rochester, Minnesota

Religious convictions, cultural attitudes, traditional customs, and personal beliefs may affect the decision of the patient proxy to proceed with organ donation. At the present time, major Western religions support organ and tissue donation (1), and only in a limited sense does objection to donation continue. The opposition may not be framed by moral objections but by the definition of death. Certain ideologies are more concerned about the afterlife and reincarnation; in others, the conversion from life to death is simply loss of breath (Hinduism) or more radically defined as decomposition (Tibetan Buddhism). There are a few contestants of brain death in Judaism and Christianity, but none of these scholars have been able to invigorate debate (see Chapter 9).

Although religious views about the concept of brain death are complex enough to attract our attention, religious affiliation is not particularly relevant for many Americans when confronted with brain death and organ donation. In addition, a considerable proportion of religious leaders are truly unaware of the concept of brain death. In 1996, a survey of 183 religious leaders in Colorado was performed. Clergy, hospital chaplains, and seminary students responded to questions about religious attitudes and organ donation and were uniformly supportive of organ donation (2).

In response to one of the statements "I believe that the declaration of brain death means that a person is dead," one of four of the respondents was "uncertain" or "believed that organ donors were not really dead at the time of donation." Only 62% of the clergy appreciated brain death as the defining departure, compared with 77% of the seminary students and 90% of the chaplains. This discrepancy between acceptance of donation of organs and uncertainty about the very moment of death reflects lack of knowledge in clergy of the central tenet of brain death despite their education.

Personal reflections associated with the sadness of brain death in a loved one bring to light religious and cultural values. This chapter focuses on a general overview of religious and cultural beliefs and how they could pertain to the acceptance of brain death and the donation process. It also examines the role of the clergy within the management team in the intensive care unit.

OVERVIEW OF RELIGIOUS BELIEFS

Many mainstream religions in the United States have official policy statements in their doctrines in support of donation. The major religions in the United States are

Christianity, Islam, and Judaism. These three religions are divided into various different denominations. Both Islam and Judaism have long traditions of defining death as the absence of respiration, but brain death has become an accepted definition of death for these religious traditions. A comprehensive discussion of the theology of death or funeral rites is outside the scope of this monograph. However, certain aspects and moral objections need attention.

With Christian denominations, the beliefs are rooted in the Bible. Jesus has told us that He is the resurrection and the life and that those who believe in him will never die. The dominant emphasis in Christianity is belief in the resurrection of Christ and his followers. Scorsone summarized in his paper on "Christianity and significance of the body" that body and soul are God's creation, but when a person dies and the soul leaves the body, organ donation should be allowed to give life to others (3). Several scriptures in the Bible may guide Christian thinking (e.g., *Luke* 6:37–38: "Give and it shall be given unto you;" *Revelation* 21:4–5: "In eternity we will not need our earthly bodies: former things will pass away, all things will be made new."). The Roman Catholic Church legitimizes organ donation by the principle of solidarity and charity.

Islam (religion of Muslims) permeates all races and requires submission to the one and only God (Allah) and His will. People have been created to worship Allah. The family system in an Islamic community is strong and includes neighbors and friends. When hardships come, the Muslim should not give up and has no right to determine anyone's time to die (to terminate support). Nonetheless, the third International Conference of Islamic Jurists was resolute in favor of defining brain death as death of a person. A person is considered legally dead, and all the Sharia's principles can be applied when one of the following signs is established:

1. Complete stoppage of the heart and breathing and the doctors decide it is irretrievable.
2. Complete stoppage of all the vital functions of the brain and the doctors decide it is irreversible and the brain has started to degenerate.

The Islamic law after death obliges shrouding the body with white cloth and a funeral prayer is offered. The body should be washed by a pious person.

The essence of Judaism is unconditional belief in God, objection to desecration of the body and delay of burial. Many different groups with different rabbinic views of the Jewish law (Halacha) exist. In the United States, orthodox, reform, conservative, reconstructionists, and secular denominations are prevalent. Orthodox Jews accept the whole Torah word for word with its restrictive traditions, but the modern orthodoxy is moderate and most people do not live secular lives. Other wings believe the Torah laws, although sacrosanct can be interpreted differently, paving the way for independence for individual congregations. Reform and Conservative Jews have accepted brain death after analysis of traditional writing by their rabbis. In contrast, Orthodox rabbis Bleich and Soloveichek in the United States and Former Chief Rabbi Lord Jakobovitz interpret the ancient teachings as cardiac arrest as the defining moment of death. An explanatory reading of the Talmudic tract published by Moses

Tendler has compared and equated brain death with decapitation and thus accepts its premise of death. The most notable act was a change in New York State legislature initiated by the Orthodox Jewish community to include a religious exemption for declaring death subjecting the physician, if ignored, to possible malpractice if death was declared (see Chapter 8). Nonetheless, the overwhelming majority of Jews support the concept of brain death. Some groups of Orthodox Jews may oppose strongly; all would need to consult with their rabbi first.

Miracles may be at the center of discussions with families because most religious traditions were founded on healing miracles. We have encountered families who have requested to pray for a healing miracle, and there have been families who gave signals to pray for a resurrection. Nothing seems more complicated.

Allan Fisher and his colleagues articulated it well:

> The unwillingness or inability to accept the reality of the death of the brain-dead patient was reflected in around 10% of the families who expressed hope that "a miracle would occur." Some were supported by the opinions of local devout leaders or healers, who would predict recovery, thereby rendering impossible any further rational discussion. Overall, when a family stated at some point that they entertained hope of recovery it was realized that organ donation was ultimately an impossibility (4).

Likewise, Christians may have faith in miracles. The Bible has examples of raising the dead through Elijah and Elisha (1 *Kings* 17; 2 *Kings* 4). However, miracles are not for the asking and Jesus, unlike other founders of religions, was generally reluctant to perform miracles. Jesus performed miracles only to make someone believe He was the Christ (*John* 20). Raising of Lazarus (from the Hebrew *Eleazar*, which means God has helped) from the dead after being entombed for days made many Jews believe in Jesus as the Christ (*John* 11).

In our experience, divine intervention creating miracles is an uncommon devotion with families. It may be desirable to discourage any such ritual. However, rather than showing skepticism, continuous communication of the hopeless situation is the best approach.

A comprehensive overview of religions and their views on organ and tissue donation is given in the Appendix. Many positions, particularly the Eastern religions, are unknown. Specific statements about a cardiocentric view of death or brain death as prerequisites for possible donation are not always available. Unless specifically stated, we cannot assume, by implication, that the definition of death is a medical issue and is to be left to the discretion of the physician.

CULTURE

Culture and religion influence and impact each other in many aspects. A person might be a Catholic and aware that the Catholic Church supports donation, but families may be from a Hispanic community that puts a great deal of emphasis on the importance of the heart. Occasionally, families may be hesitant to donate their loved one's heart, but would allow the donation of other organs.

Data provided by the United Network of Organ Sharing (UNOS) on ethnicity in donors consistently shows a persistent trend of African-American, Hispanic, and Asian rates below that of whites. A fact is that organ donation is much less approved among different racial groups (9). Some believe it is due to poor understanding, education, or mistrust of the messenger (6). Barriers that complicate the decision to donate may include lack of faith in success of transplantation, hostility toward physicians, or problems with communication.

African-Americans usually are from religious traditions such as Baptist or Methodist that are very supportive of donation. However, perceived experiences of being mistreated by the medical community may influence decisions on donation (8). There are a few that feel African-American donors are not needed and fear that whites are more helped than blacks by donation. African-Americans do have a mistrust in many surveys and in one survey often agreed with the statement, "Doctors would not try as hard to save me if they knew I was an organ donor" (7). Callender championed much of the organ donor campaigns in the African-American community and identified five common reasons for unwillingness to donate in the black population of the District of Columbia. First, there is a documented lack of awareness of renal disease and transplantation. Second, religious myths, misperceptions, and superstitions prevail among all income levels. Third, trust in health care providers and the health administrative process is fragile and evident in many interactions with families. Fourth, there is a perception that the signing of an organ donor card might change the emphasis from life saving to organ donor priority. Finally, there is a perceived fear that racism, which African-Americans experience on a daily basis in life, would remain after death, resulting in all black donated organs going to white people (9,10). Moreover, many minorities, especially African-Americans, wait twice as long for kidneys as do whites. This is a result of HLA typing during allocation and difficulty with finding matches between races. This longer waiting time has been misinterpreted as racial prejudice by some. Despite the prevailing sense in some African-Americans that organ donation is not fair, nine out of ten African-Americans receive a graft from a white donor.

Similar apprehension may be seen in tribes of the Native Americans. Most Native Americans believe in a "Creator or Master Spirit." However, Native American cultures are wary of organ donation, based on their spiritual beliefs of the afterlife. Organ donation is a concern of great debate in these communities, but no official position is known. Reservations in the upper Midwest with traditional Pow Wows showed increased willingness when approached by similar health care workers of their culture. Another survey identified hesitation prompted by the possibility of donating their unhealthy organs but also a desire to keep the body intact (11). Here again the pietistic role of the body comes into play.

Hispanic population encompassing people of Mexican, Puerto Rican, and Cuban heritage cite mutilation of the body as a common concern. Some immigrants from the Caribbean countries do believe disturbing the body may anger the spirit of the body. How much of these superstitions permeate in the Hispanic community is unknown, but they are unlikely to be the norm (12).

Roma ("gypsies") are a people of a distinct ethnicity with a set of folk beliefs. Virtually all oppose organ and tissue donation. Approximately 12 million Romani live in Europe, Russia, and the Middle East. Traditional belief contends that, for 1 year after death, the soul retraces its steps. The soul maintains its physical shape, and the body must remain intact. Many Roma adopt the faith of the countries they reside in, including Roman Catholicism, Eastern Orthodox, and Islamic religions. Strong family traditions exist, and families may create clans. Roma believe in healing rituals and practice fortune telling and supernatural ways to cure disease. After death, some Roma believe evil spirits can enter the body, which is reflected by a desire to plug the nostrils with wax or pearls (13).

Many other cults and spiritual movements, prevalent in China, have not expressed any opinions on brain death, largely because these disciplines seek other priorities. The Japanese attitude and its complex history has been recounted in Chapter 1.

All these cultural attitudes, superstitions, and prejudices may be separate from their original religious beliefs and negatively impact on care, brain death acceptance, and possible organ procurement. Regardless of the race, cultural background, or religion of the health care team, it is imperative to approach the family in a manner that is sensitive to their culture and religion. Education and awareness of minorities has been greatly enhanced by task forces and the "National Minority Donor Awareness Day." Dr. Cass Franklin, chairman of the UNOS minority affairs committee, stated in December 10, 1996, that "with regard to extrarenal transplantation (liver, hearts . . .) we have not demonstrated any ethnic inequities in the allocation or distribution of organs" (www.unos.org/newsroom). The problems at the recipient end in minorities remain formidable.

ROLE OF THE CLERGY

Clergy can play a crucial role in the mediation between family and physician and it is important to be able to view them as supportive but neutral allies.

Some hospitals entrust the request for donation with the hospital chaplain, but chaplains do not have consent rates as high as trained organ procurement coordinators. As was mentioned earlier, many religious leaders do not fully understand the concept of brain death and may confuse it with other comatose states such as a vegetative state. When a family is divided, the chaplain can explain the major benefits of organ donation, try to heal mistrust, if any, and explain the urgency of the decision.

Hospital chaplains can be instrumental in offering final praying or last rites. It can be difficult for family members, as well as clergy and medical personnel, to fully realize the finality of brain death. Having specific prayers and other "good-bye" rituals said at the bedside can be very comforting.

CLERGY EDUCATION

There are many additional avenues for clergy education besides inclusion in curriculum. National Donor Sabbath (NDS) is focused on religion. The National Donor Sabbath as part of a national organ and donor initiative premiered in 1998 with the support of Vice President Al Gore and Secretary of Health Donna Shalala to promote organ donation through clergy. National Organ and Tissue Donor Awareness Week (NOTDAW) is targeted at the general public. Both are yearly events which can reach out to clergy and to help the general public understand their religious tradition and its views on donation. National Donor Sabbath is typically two weekends before Thanksgiving and is an interfaith time for congregations to come together around the subject of life and thanksgiving. NOTDAW is often near the Christian holiday of Easter and the Jewish celebration of Passover. Springtime themes of renewal and new life can be used with all religions.

Clergy can, in turn, educate their congregations via sermons, literature, and other forms of education. UNOS has issued a comprehensive guide for clergy which contains several examples of sermons (*Organ and Tissue Donation: A Reference Guide for Clergy*, 3rd ed., 2000). One sermon can be a powerful statement in support of organ donation from a source that is seen as neutral, understanding, trustworthy, and knowledgeable. Seminaries need to begin incorporating organ donation and brain death into their pastoral care classes. Hospital chaplain programs such as clinical pastoral education (CPE) also need to clearly focus on this subject.

Yet another possibility for clergy education is through the incorporation of seminars and doctor–clergy breakfasts which are currently held at some hospitals. This is an opportunity for physicians and religious leaders to become familiar with these topics and enhance educational dialogue and partnership.

RELIGIOUS CONFLICT RESOLUTION

Religion and spirituality affect the greater part of the American public and other societies but rarely fully determines the decision to donate organs and tissue. The reasons for refusal involve private beliefs, possible concern about disfigurement, but most commonly unfamiliarity of the proxy with the prior wishes of the brain-dead person (see Chapter 10). When religious or cultural objections are put forward by the family members, it is important to have families hold a conference with their own minister, priest, or religious leader. In our experience, local pastors have been very helpful in clarification of brain death and the process of donation. It is important to emphasize that organ donation can save many lives, not just one.

Some families question whether an incomplete body may go to heaven or preclude resurrection. Some people cite that God has promised to make all things whole in death. To resolve this matter, we have emphasized that many persons die by fire or destructive accidents and cremations are commonly performed. Nonetheless, fringe religions and cultural beliefs may object to the determination of brain death and express a desire to try all possible care. Typically, all available options are requested, including pharmaceutical support, prolonged cardiac resuscitation, and continuous stay in the ICU with comprehensive nursing care. Ethical committees in consultation may be useful, but ambivalence and discomfort will remain with the attending physician. In certain cases, transfer of the patient to another hospital may be considered (see Chapter 8) but will probably rarely be successful. When no resolution can be achieved, continuation of care (but anticipating cardiac arrest) is probably the only option.

CONCLUSION

There is support from Western and Eastern religions for both organ donation and the concept of brain death, particularly in Christians and increasingly in Jews and Muslims (88–90). Although initially expected otherwise, ultra-conservative Christian denominations have made a very strong statement in favor of organ donation. The main impediment is that many religious leaders and their congregants are unaware of this support and lack some degree of medical knowledge. Opposition in some orthodox Jewish groups remains. In many religions the concern of desecration of the body after death is overridden by the obligation to save lives by organ donation. By combining efforts with physicians and OPOs, clergy may contribute to increase the number of organ donors around the world.

APPENDIX: RELIGIOUS VIEWS ON ORGAN/TISSUE DONATION AND TRANSPLANTATION

AME and AME Zion (African Methodist Episcopal)

This is a Protestant denomination that is made up primarily of African-American members. Organ and tissue donation is viewed as an act of neighborly love and charity by these denominations. They encourage all members to support donation as a way of helping others.

Amish

The Amish will consent to transplantation if they believe it is for the well-being of the transplant recipient. John Hostetler, world renowned authority on Amish religion and Professor of Anthropology at Temple University in Philadelphia, says in his book, *Amish Society,* "The Amish believe that since God created the human body, it is God who heals. However, nothing in the Amish understanding of the Bible forbids them from using modern medical services, including surgery, hospitalization, dental work, anesthesia, blood transfusions or immunization."

Assembly of God

Assembly of God is an independent Protestant Christian denomination. The Church has no official policy regarding organ and tissue donation, but the decision to donate is left to the individual. Donation is highly supported by the denomination.

Baptist

There are a variety of Protestant Baptist denominations. Donation is supported as an act of charity and the church leaves the decision to donate to the individual.

Brethren

Another Protestant denomination, The Church of the Brethren's Annual Conference in 1993 developed a resolution on organ and tissue donation supporting and encouraging donation. They stated, "We have the opportunity to help others out of love for Christ, through the donation of organs and tissues" (14).

Buddhism

Buddhism originated in Asia, but there are also a number of Buddhists in the United States. Buddhists believe that organ or tissue donation is a matter of individual conscience and place high value on acts of compassion. Reverend Gyomay Masao, President and Founder of the Buddhist Temple of Chicago, says, "We honor those people who donate their bodies and organs to the advancement of medical science and to saving lives." The importance of letting loved ones know your wishes is stressed. However, many families will not give permission to donate unless they know their loved one's preferences (15–22).

Catholicism

Catholics view organ or tissue donation as an act of charity and love, and the Pope has been outspoken in his support of donation. Pope John Paul II stated in an address to the Society For Organ Sharing 1991, "With the advent of organ transplantation, which began with blood transfusion, man has found a way to give of himself, of his blood and of his body, so that others may continue to live . . . The medical act of transplantation makes possible the donor's act of self-giving, that sincere gift of self which expresses our constitutive calling to love and communion" (23–26). A more recent address to the 18th International Congress of the Transplantation Society (August 29, 2000) specifically mentioned brain death:

> It is a well-known fact that for some time certain scientific approaches to ascertaining death have shifted the emphasis from the traditional cardiorespiratory signs to the so-called "neurological" criterion. Specifically, this consists in establishing, according to clearly determined parameters commonly held by the international scientific community, the complete and irreversible cessation of all brain activity (in the cerebrum, cerebellum and brain stem). This is then considered the sign that the individual organism has lost its integrative capacity.

Christian Church (Disciples of Christ)

This Protestant denomination encourages organ and tissue donation, stating that individuals were created for God's glory and for sharing God's love. A 1985 resolution, adopted by the general assembly, encourages "members of the Christian Church (Disciples of Christ) to enroll as organ donors and prayerfully support those who have received an organ transplant" (27–30).

Christian Science

The Church of Christ Scientist does not have a specific position regarding organ and tissue donation. According to the First Church of Christ Scientist in Boston, Christian Scientists normally rely on spiritual means of healing instead of medical. They are free, however, to choose whatever form of medical treatment they desire — including a transplant. The question of organ or tissue donation is an individual decision.

Episcopal

The Episcopal Church passed a resolution in 1982 that recognizes the life-giving benefits of organ, blood, and tissue donation. All Christians are encouraged to become organ, blood, and tissue donors "as part of their ministry to others in the name of Christ, who gave His life that we may have life in its fullness."

Greek Orthodox

According to Reverend Dr. Milton Efthimiou, Director of the Department of Church and Society for the Greek Orthodox Church of North and South America, "the Greek Orthodox Church is not opposed to organ donation as long as the organs and tissue in question are used to better human life, i.e., for transplantation or for research that will lead to improvements in the treatment and prevention of disease."

Hinduism

According to the Hindu Temple Society of North America, Hindus are not prohibited by religious law from donating their organs. This act is an individual's decision. H.L. Trivedi stated that, "Hindu mythology has stories in which the parts of the human body are used for the benefit of other humans and society. There is nothing in the Hindu religion indicating that parts of humans, dead or alive, cannot be used to alleviate the suffering of other humans" (81–85).

Independent Conservative Evangelical

Generally, Evangelical Protestants have no opposition to organ and tissue donation. Each church is autonomous and leaves the decision to donate to the individual.

Islam

The religion of Islam strongly believes in the principle of saving human lives. The Qu'ran says about charity "and whosoever saves a human life is as though he has saved all mankind." According to A. Sachedina, "the majority of the Muslim scholars belonging to various schools of Islamic law have invoked the principle of priority of saving human life and have permitted the organ transplant as a necessity to procure that noble end." The Islamic code of medical ethics states the donation of body fluids or organs is "*Farah kitaya*," a duty that donors fulfill on behalf of society. The Academy of Islamic Jurisprudence declared acceptance of the concept of brain death (31–44).

Jehovah's Witnesses

According to their National Headquarters, the Watch Tower Society, Jehovah's Witnesses believe donation is a matter of individual decision. Jehovah's Witnesses are often assumed to be opposed to donation because of their belief against blood transfusion. However, this merely means that all blood must be removed from the organs and tissues before being transplanted. In addition, it would not be acceptable for an organ donor to receive blood as part of the organ recovery process (45,46).

Judaism

All four branches of Judaism (Orthodox, Conservative, Reform, and Reconstructionist) support and encourage donation. According to Orthodox Rabbi Moses Tendler, Chairman of the Biology Department of Yeshiva University in New York City and chairman of the Bioethics Commission of the Rabbinical Council of America, "If one is in the position to donate an organ to save another's life, it's obligatory to do so, even if the donor never knows who the beneficiary will be. The basic principle of Jewish ethics—'the infinite worth of the human being'—also includes donation of corneas, since eyesight restoration is considered a life-saving operation." In 1991, the Rabbinical Council of America (Orthodox) approved organ donations as permissible, even required, from brain-dead patients. Both the Reform and Conservative movements also have policy statements strongly supporting donation (47–69).

Lutheran

In 1984, the Lutheran Church in America (Missouri Synod) passed a resolution stating that donation contributes to the well-being of humanity and can be "an expression of sacrificial love for a neighbor in need." They call on "members to consider donating organs and to make any necessary family and legal arrangements, including the use of a signed donor card." They are one of the largest Protestant denominations in the United States (70–72).

Mennonite

Mennonites are a Protestant denomination with no formal position on donation, but are not opposed to it. They believe the decision to donate is up to the individual and their family.

Mormon (Church of Jesus Christ of Latter-Day Saints)

According to Lester E. Bush, Jr., in his 1993 book, *Health and Medicine among the Latter-Day Saints,* Mormons have recently described donation "as an act of 'selfless love,' and notable transplant successes among members are publicized in church periodicals." Officially, it is noted that the decision to donate is an individual one made in conjunction with family, medical personnel, and prayer (72,73).

Moravian

The Moravian Church does not have an official policy addressing organ/tissue donation or transplantation. Robert E. Sawyer, President, Provincial Elders Conference, Moravian Church of America, Southern Province, states, "There is nothing in our doctrine or policy that would prevent a Moravian pastor from assisting a family in making a decision to donate or not to donate an organ." It is, therefore, a matter of individual choice (74).

Orthodox Christian

Reverend Victor Sokolov notes that "There is nothing in our Church's doctrine prohibiting the donation of needed organs after a person's death. On the contrary, the Lord enthusiastically approves the laying down of one's life for his friends (John 15:13). He would surely welcome the sharing of organs no longer needed with those whose lives could be prolonged and saved."

Presbyterian

Presbyterians encourage and support donation and are a large Protestant denomination in the United States. They respect a person's right to make decisions regarding their own body. During their General Assembly in 1995, they stated a strong support of donation and commented that they "encourage its members and friends to sign and carry Universal Donor Cards . . . "

Seventh-Day Adventist

Donation and transplantation are strongly encouraged by Seventh-Day Adventists. They have many transplant hospitals, including Loma Linda in California. Loma Linda specializes in pediatric heart transplantation.

Shinto

Shinto is a folk religion found in Japan. In Shinto, the dead body is considered to be impure and dangerous, and thus quite powerful. "In folk belief context, injuring a dead body is a serious crime . . ." according to E. Namihira in his article, "Shinto Concept Concerning the Dead Human Body." "To this day it is difficult to obtain consent from bereaved families for organ donation or dissection for medical education or pathological anatomy . . . the Japanese practicing Shinto regard them all in the sense of injuring a dead body." Families are often concerned that they not injure the *itai*— the relationship between the dead person and the bereaved people (75,76).

Society of Friends (Quaker)

Organ and tissue donation is believed to be an individual decision. The Society of Friends does not have an official position on donation.

Unitarian Universalist

Unitarian Universalists affirm the inherent worth and dignity of every person and respect the interdependent web of all existence. They affirm the value of organ and tissue donation, but leave the decision to each individual.

United Church of Christ

Reverend Jay Litner, Director, Washington Office of the United Church of Christ Office for Church in Society, states that "United Church of Christ people, churches and agencies are extremely and overwhelmingly supportive of organ sharing. The General Synod has never spoken to this issue because, in general, the Synod speaks on more controversial issues, and there is no controversy about organ sharing, just as there is no controversy about blood donation in the denomination. While the General Synod has never spoken about blood donation, blood donation rooms have been set up at several General Synods. Similarly, any organized effort to get the General Synod delegates or individual churches to sign organ donation cards would meet with generally positive responses."

United Methodist

The United Methodist Church issued a policy statement in 1984 regarding organ and tissue donation. In it, they state that "The United Methodist Church recognizes the life-giving benefits of organ and tissue donation, and thereby encourages all Christians to become organ and tissue donors by signing and carrying cards or driver's licenses, attesting to their commitment of such organs upon their death, to those in need, as part of their ministry to others in the name of Christ, who gave his life that we might have life in its fullness." A 1992 resolution states, "Donation is to be encouraged, assuming appropriate safeguards against hastening death and determination of death by reliable criteria." The resolution further states that, "Pastoral-care persons should be willing to explore these options as a normal part of conversation with patients and their families" (77–79).

Wesleyan Church

The Wesleyan Church supports donation as a way of helping others. They believe that God's "ability to resurrect us is not dependent on whether or not all our parts were connected at death." They also support research and in 1989 noted in a task force on public morals and social concerns that "one of the ways that a Christian can do good is to request that their body be donated to a medical school for use in teaching" (80).

ACKNOWLEDGMENTS

The appendix was originally compiled by Christine Gallagher. Policy position statements from various religious denominations have also been obtained by Charles H. Chandler, D.Min., UNOS clergy consultant. An adapted appendix was published in *Organ and Tissue Donation: A Reference Guide for Clergy,* edited by M. Lisa Cooper Hammon and Gloria J. Taylor (2000, SEOPF/UNOS), and parts have been reproduced with permission.

REFERENCES

1. De Long WR, ed. *Organ transplantation in religious, ethical and social context—no room for death.* New York: Haworth Pastoral Press, 1993.
2. Gallagher C. Religious attitudes regarding organ donation. *J Transplant Coord* 1996;6:186–190.
3. Scorsone S. Christianity and significance of the human body. *Transplant Proc* 1990;22:943–944.
4. Fisher A, Herzog LJ, Herzog EM. Five years' experience of an organ donation team in southern Israel. *Isr J Med Sci* 1996;32:1112–1119.
5. Fins JA. Across the divide: religious objections to brain death. *J Religion Health* 1995;34:33–39.
6. Wheeler MS, Cheung AH. Minority attitudes toward organ donation. *Crit Care Nurse* 1996; 16:30–35.
7. Yuen CC, Burton W, Chiraseveenuprapund D, et al. Attitudes and beliefs about organ donation among different racial groups. *J Natl Med Assoc* 1998;90:13–18.
8. Wheeler MS, O'Friel M, Cheung AHS, et al. Cultural beliefs of Asian Americans as barriers to organ donation. *J Transplant Coord* 1994;4:146–150.
9. Callender CO, Bey A. A national minority organ/tissue transplant education program. *Transplant Proc* 1995;27:1441–1443.
10. Callender CO, Hall LE, Yeager CL, et al. Organ donation and Blacks. A critical frontier. *N Engl J Med* 1991;325:442–444.
11. Blagg CR, Helgerson SD, Warren CW, et al. Awareness and attitiudes of Northwest Native Americans regarding organ donation and transplantation. *Clin Transplant* 1992;46:436–442.
12. Ciancio G, Burke GW, Gomez C, et al. Organ donation among Hispanics: a single-center experience. *Transplant Proc* 1997;29:3745.
13. Yoors J. *Gypsies.* Waveland Press, 1987.
14. Resolution on Organ and Tissue Donation. Presented at the Church of the Brethren Annual Conference, Indianapolis, June 22–27, 1993.
15. Bhikkhu, Venerable Mettanando. Buddhist ethics in the practice of medicine. In: Wei-hsun Fu C, Wawrytko SA, eds. *Buddhist Ethics and Modern Society: An International Symposium.* 195–213.
16. Fujii M. Buddhism and bioethics. In: Lustig BA, et al., eds. *Bioethics yearbook. Vol. 1: Theological developments in bioethics, 1988–1990.* Boston: Kluwer Academic, 1991:66–67.
17. Green J. Death with dignity: Buddhism. *Nurs Times* 1989;85:40–41.
18. Hardacre H. Response of Buddhism and Shinto to the issue of brain death and organ transplant. *Camb Q Healthcare Ethics* 1994;3:585–601.
19. Keyes CD, Wisest WE, eds. Introduction to religious perspectives: Buddhism. In: *New Harvest: Transplanting body parts and reaping the benefits.* Clifton, NJ: Humana Press, 1991:184–185.
20. Lecso PA. The Bodhisattva ideal and organ transplantation. *J Religion Health* 1991;30:35–40.
21. Sugunasiri SHJ. The Buddhist view concerning the dead body. *Transplant Proc* 1990;22; 947–949.
22. Tsuji KT. The Buddhist view of the body and organ transplantation. *Transplant Proc* 1988; 20:1076–1078.
23. *Ethical and religious directives for Catholic health care facilities,* rev. ed. Washington, DC: U.S. Catholic Conference, Office of Publishing and Promotion Services, 1975.
24. Green J. Death with dignity: Roman Catholicism. *Nurs Times* 1992;88:26–27.
25. Keyes CD, Wiest WE, eds. Introduction to religious perspectives: Roman Catholic interpretation. In: *New harvest: transplanting body parts and reaping the benefits.* Clifton, NJ: Humana Press, 1991:199–211.
26. Teo B. Organ donation and transplantation: a Christian viewpoint. *Transplant Proc* 1992; 24.2114–2115.
27. Green J. Death with dignity: Christian science. *Nurs Times* 1992;88:32–33.
28. Harakas SS. Eastern Orthodox bioethics. In: Lustig BA, et al., eds. *Bioethics yearbook. Vol. 1: Theological developments in bioethics, 1988–1990.* Boston: Kluwer Academic, 1991:97.
29. Harakas SS. *Health and medicine in the Eastern Orthodox tradition.* New York: Crossroad Publishing, 1990:156–159.
30. Harakas SS. *Living the faith: the praxis of Eastern Orthodox ethics.* Minneapolis: Light and Life Publishing, 1992.
31. Al-Mousawi M, Hamed T, al-Matouk H. Views of Muslim scholars on organ donation and brain death. *Transplant Proc* 1997;29:3217.
32. Aswad S. The role of public education in cadaveric transplantation in Saudi Arabia. *Transplant Proc* 1991;23:2694–2696.
33. Egypt's two highest Islamic authorities clash over Moslem's right to donate organs. *Transplant News* 1995 Aug 28:7.
34. Green J. Death with dignity: Islam. *Nurs Times* 1989;85:56–57.

35. Hassaballah AM. Definition of death, organ donation and interruption of treatment in Islam. *Nephrol Dial Transplant* 1996;11:964–965.
36. Hathout H. Islamic concepts and bioethics. In: Lustig BA, et al., eds. *Bioethics yearbook. Vol. 1: Theological developments in bioethics, 1988–1990.* Boston: Kluwer Academic, 1991:114–115.
37. Indonesian Muslims to issue fatwa allowing kidney transplants. *Transplant News* 1996 May 28:5.
38. Keyes CD, Wiest WE, eds. Introduction to religious perspectives: Islam. In: *New Harvest: Transplanting body parts and reaping the benefits.* Clifton, NJ: Humana Press, 1991:181–182.
39. Moslem Law Council issues decree allowing British Moslems to donate organs. *Transplant News* 1995 Aug 28:7.
40. Palmer AI. The Islamic ruling on brain death and life support. www.Islaam.com. 2000 April 30:1–4.
41. Rasheed HZA. Organ donation and transplantation—a Muslim viewpoint. *Transplant Proc* 1992; 24:2116–2117.
42. Sachedina AA. Islamic views on organ transplantation. *Transplant Proc* 1988;20:1084–1088.
43. Sahin AF. Islamic transplantation ethics. *Transplant Proc* 1990;22:939.
44. Sellami MM. Islamic position on organ donation and transplantation. *Transplant Proc* 1993; 25:2307–2309.
45. Mallory GB Jr. Challenging issues associated with organ transplantation for Jehovah's Witness individual. *J Heart Lung Transplant* 2000;19:119–120.
46. Watch Tower Bible and Tract Society of Pennsylvania. *How can blood save your life?* New York: Watchtower Bible and Tract Society of New York, 1990.
47. Berkowitz AK. Jews and organ donations: all take and no give? *Moment Mag* 1995 Aug:32–35,58–59.
48. Blech JD. *Judaism and healing: Halakhic perspectives.* KTAV Publishing House.
49. Breitowitz, Rabbi Yitzchok. The brain death controversy in Jewish law. www.jlaw.com. 2000 April 30:1–3.
50. Bulka RP. Jewish perspective on organ transplantation. *Transplant Proc* 1990;22:945–946.
51. Camenisch P. *Religious methods and resources in bioethics.* London: Kluwer Academic Publishers, 1994.
52. Dobrusin, Rabbi Robert. Organ donation in Jewish law. www.hvcn.org/info/bethisrael/rabbi/organs.html. 1996 June 24:1–2.
53. Gerson B. Transplantation: a Jewish perspective. *Intermountain Jewish News* 1995 Nov.
54. Goldman AL. Religion notes: ruling on transplants. *New York Times* 1991 June 15:10.
55. Green J. Death with dignity: Judaism. *Nurs Times* 1989;85:64–65.
56. Inwald D, Jakobovits I, Petros A. Brainstem death: managing care when accepting medical guidelines and religious beliefs are in conflict. Consideration and compromise are possible. *BMJ* 2000;320:1266–1267.
57. Keyes CD, Wiest WE, eds. Introduction to religious perspectives: Jewish perspectives. In: *New harvest: transplanting body parts and reaping the benefits.* Clifton, NJ: Humana Press, 1991:187–197.
58. Neuman I. Rabbi, doctor, transplant coordinator Issack Neuman converts Jews to principles of donation. *UNOS Update* 1995 Nov:18,22.
59. Olick RS. Brain death, religious freedom, and public policy: New Jersey's landmark legislative initiative. *Kennedy Inst Ethics J* 1991;1:275–288.
60. Organ and tissue donation: the gift of life, the Conservative Jewish position. Presented at the Federation of Jewish Men's Clubs Mid Atlantic Region, 1990.
61. Pearl AJ. Get yourself a new heart: Judaism and the organ transplantation issue. *Can Med Assoc J* 1990;143:1365–1367.
62. Rabbi rules ultra-Orthodox Jews can donate their organs as long as it's to other Jews. *Transplant News* 1996 April 28:6.
63. Rappaport ZH, Isabelle T. Principles and concepts of brain death and organ donation: the Jewish perspective. *Childs Nerv Syst* 1998;14:381–383.
64. Rosenbluth SL. Organ transplant: soon it may be a routine part of the Jewish death ritual. *Jewish Voice Opin* 1996 Dec.
65. Rosner F. *Modern medicine and Jewish law.* New York: Yeshiva University, Department of Special Publications, 1972.
66. Rosner F. *Studies in Torah Judaism: modern medicine and Jewish law.* New York: Balshon Printing and Offset, 1972.
67. Sebert LA. The gift of life. *Jewish Week* 1995 Sept 15:22–23.
68. Steinberg A. Judaism and bioethics. In: Lustig BA, et al., eds. *Bioethics yearbook. Vol. 1: Theological developments in bioethics, 1988–1990.* Boston: Kluwer Academic, 1991:193–194.
69. Weiss DW. Religious and cultural issues: organ transplantation, medical ethics, and Jewish law. *Transplant Proc* 1988;20:1071–1075.

70. Lustig BA. Bioethics in the Lutheran tradition. In: Lustig BA, et al., eds. *Bioethics yearbook. Vol. 1: Theological developments in bioethics, 1988–1990.* Boston: Kluwer Academic, 1991:139.
71. The Lutheran Church–Missouri Synod. *Resolution 8-05. To Encourage Donation of Kidneys and Other Organs.*
72. Campbell CS. The Latter-Day Saints and medical ethics. In: Lustig BA, et al., eds. *Bioethics yearbook. Vol. 1: Theological developments in bioethics, 1988–1990.* Boston: Kluwer Academic, 1991:36–38.
73. Green J. Death with dignity: the Mormon Church. *Nurs Times* 1992;88:44–45.
74. Sokolov, Reverend Victor. Death, funeral, requiem—Orthodox Christian traditions, customs and practice. www.holy-trinity.org/liturgics/sokolov-death.html. 2000 April 30:1–4.
75. Hardacre H. Response of Buddhism and Shinto to the issue of brain death and organ transplant. *Camb Q Healthcare Ethics* 1994;3:585–601.
76. Namihira E. Shinto concept concerning the dead human body. *Transplant Proc* 1990;22:940–941.
77. Shelton RT. Organ donation and transplantation. In: Lustig BA, et al., eds. *Bioethics yearbook, Vol. 1: Theological developments in bioethics, 1988–1990.* Boston: Kluwer Academic, 1991:158.
78. United Methodist Church. *The book of resolutions of the United Methodist Church.* Nashville, TN: The United Methodist Publishing House, 1984.
79. United Methodist Church. *The book of resolutions of the United Methodist Church.* Nashville, TN: The United Methodist Publishing House, 1992.
80. Wesleyan Church, Task Force on Public Morals and Social Concerns. *Position paper on issues related to death and dying.* Indianapolis: Wesleyan Church, 1989.
81. Ethical considerations in xenotransplantation. In: *A new wave in transplantation—catch it!* St. Petersburg Beach, FL: LifeLink and Bayfront Medical Center, 1993.
82. Green J. Death with dignity: Hinduism. *Nurs Times* 1989;85:50–51.
83. Kahan BD. Ganesha: the primeval Hindu xenograft. *Transplant Proc* 1989;21:1–8.
84. Keyes CD, Wiest WE, eds. Introduction to religious perspectives: Hinduism. In: *New harvest: transplanting body parts and reaping the benefits.* Clifton, NJ: Humana Press, 1991:182–183.
85. Trivedi HL. Hindu religious view in context of transplantation of organs from cadavers. *Transplant Proc* 1990;22:942.
86. Ebersole M. *Medical ethics, human choices.* Scottsdale, PA: Herald Press, 1988.
87. Green J. Death with dignity: Christianity. *Nurs Times* 1992;88:26–27.
88. Keyes CD, Wiest WE, eds. Introduction to religious perspectives: Christian perspectives. In: *New harvest: transplanting body parts and reaping the benefits.* Clifton, NJ: Humana Press, 1991:210–221.
89. May WF. Religious justifications for donating body parts. *Hastings Cent Rep* 1985;15:38–42.
90. Thomasma DC. The quest for organ donors: a theological response. *Health Prog* 1988 Sept:22–28.

8

Legal Aspects of Brain Death

H. Richard Beresford

Cornell University Law School, University of Rochester School of Medicine, Ithaca, New York

Today laws in the United States permit physicians to diagnose death based on irreversible loss of functions of the brain. Although there is some variation in the laws of individual states, the differences are for the most part insignificant. That death occurs when the brain has ceased to function is widely accepted—provided that examining physicians apply generally accepted clinical criteria in determining that relevant brain functions are permanently lost (see Chapters 4 and 5). The emphasis of the laws is on quantitative assessment. A function is either present or absent, and the absence of function is either reversible or irreversible. Qualitative concerns, such as the dismal current predicament of a grievously brain-injured person, his or her poor prospects for later sentience, or the stresses on family members, are not a formal part of the assessment. Moreover, it falls to presumptively expert clinicians—not family or other interested parties—to make the "technical" and final determination that brain functions are absent and irreversibly so.

The existence of a legal consensus about brain death has not quelled all controversy. Residual moral and ethical concerns continue to surface (see Chapter 9). These include an unease about the seeming instrumental bias of formulating a "new" definition of death so as to facilitate organ transplantation, or about possible expansions of the definition of brain death to encompass persistent vegetative states or other forms of profound cognitive impairment. Clinical or technical concerns persist as well. They center on risks of diagnostic error, or on the lack of expertise of some clinicians who may be called on to determine brain death. There are also individuals and institutions who on theological or other principled grounds reject the very concept that death occurs at the moment the brain ceases to function. Aside from these concerns of policy and principle, clinicians have become entangled in legal disputes about the accuracy of determinations of brain death, or deriving from the ways in which they have handled relationships with families of individuals diagnosed as dead by neurological criteria.

In light of these lingering concerns, this chapter will attend to several legal and policy issues relating to brain death. After an account of the formal legal status of brain death, ensuing sections will address legal aspects of errors in diagnosis or management of brain death, legal overtones of conceptual disagreements about brain death, and legal precedents that bear on potential attempts to expand the definition of brain death beyond its current limits. The focus will be on laws of the United States. This undoubtedly limits the value of the chapter for readers who reside outside the United States. But many of the legal and policy issues arising under U.S. law are generic in the sense they are likely to emerge in a similar form in any legal system that allows for the possibility of determining death by reference to the status of brain function. For example, although brain death in the United Kingdom is determined by reference only to brainstem functions, legally oriented discussions that might arise about standards or criteria for determining loss of brain function, errors in diagnosis, validity of the concept of brain death, and slippery slopes to an expanded definition of death seem parallel to those that might ensue in the U.S.

BRAIN DEATH IN THE UNITED STATES: FORMAL LEGAL STATUS

Death as Legally Significant Event

The fact and time of a person's death have obvious legal implications. Insurance proceeds may become payable. Wills and non-testamentary transfers become subject to probate proceedings and ultimate implementation. Claims for malpractice or wrongful death, or criminal prosecutions for homicide may be triggered. Of special relevance to brain death, organs of the deceased may become available for transplantation. For these and other reasons, therefore, lawmakers have an important stake in how death is defined and determined. Although lawmakers ordinarily leave to physicians the matter of deciding when death has occurred, they have asserted the power to require physicians to adhere to a particular standard for determining death, such as irreversible cessation of all brain or cardiorespiratory functions. Thus, a physician who believes that an individual who is permanently unconscious but not ventilator-dependent is dead would risk criminal prosecution or a civil claim for wrongful death if he or she acted on this belief. As the Washington state supreme court observed in 1980, "law has independent interests in defining death which may be lost when deference to medicine is complete" (1).

Brain Death Legislation

The basis for most brain death laws in the United States is the Uniform Determination of Death Act (UDDA) (2). It provides that a person is dead if there is "irreversible cessation" of either circulatory and respiratory functions, or "all functions of the entire brain, including the brain stem." The only proviso is that the determination must be made "in accordance with accepted medical standards." In short, under the UDDA a person is dead when physicians determine, by applying prevailing clinical criteria, that cardiorespiratory or brain functions are absent and cannot be retrieved. The UDDA has been adopted by 31 states and the District of Columbia (Table 8-1), and 13 additional states have accepted the basic elements of the UDDA in formulating their brain death statutes (3). Two states, Alabama (4) and West Virginia (5), have adopted the Uniform Brain Death Act (UBDA) (6). It provides that for "legal and

TABLE 8-1. *Uniform Determination of Death Act (UDDA)*

Text of act: "An individual who has sustained either (1) irreversible cessation of circulatory and respiratory functions, or (2) irreversible cessation of all functions of the entire brain, including the brainstem, is dead. A determination of death must be made in accordance with accepted medical standards."

Jurisdictions that are adopting UDDA: Arkansas, California, Colorado, Delaware, District of Columbia, Georgia, Idaho, Indiana, Kansas, Maine, Maryland, Michigan, Minnesota, Mississippi, Missouri, Montana, Nebraska, Nevada, New Hampshire, New Mexico, North Dakota, Ohio, Oklahoma, Oregon, Pennsylvania, Rhode Island, South Carolina, South Dakota, Utah, Vermont, West Virginia, and Wyoming.

From Uniform Determination of Death Act, 12 *Uniform Laws Annotated* 589 (West 1993 and West Supp 1997).

---

medical purposes" an individual is dead if "all functions of the brain, including the brain stem," have irreversibly ceased, and the determination is made "in accordance with reasonable medical standards."

Two statutory modifications of the basic theme are of interest. The Virginia brain death statute aims to enhance reliability of clinical determinations by spelling out that there be "the absence of brain stem reflexes, spontaneous brain functions and spontaneous respiratory functions" before death is determined, and requiring that the physician making this determination be "a specialist in the field of neurology, neurosurgery, or electroencephalography" (7). The New Jersey brain death statute, while permitting use of "neurological criteria" to determine death, specifically forbids use of such criteria if a physician has "reason to believe . . . that such a declaration would violate the personal religious beliefs of the individual" (8). The appendix to this chapter provides a state-by-state tabulation of statutes, regulations or judicial decisions that currently provide the legal authority for determination of death by neurological criteria.

Judicial Decisions

In several states whose legislatures have not yet enacted brain death statutes, the highest courts have ruled that it is lawful to determine death based on irreversible loss of all brain functions (1,9–11) (see Appendix). These rulings have been made in the context of a murder trial in which a defendant asserted that removal of a ventilator from a putatively "brain-dead" patient was the cause of death, not the defendant's allegedly homicidal conduct, leaving a modest residual uncertainty about applicability in other legal settings (12). One state, New York, has responded by issuing health department regulations that codify the definition of death set forth in the Uniform Determination of Death Act and authorize health care providers to determine death on the basis of neurological criteria (13). These regulations also mandate notification of next of kin or other significant persons before such criteria are applied so as to allow for a "reasonable accommodation" to "religious or moral objections" to use of the criteria in making a clinical determination of death.

Constraints on Applying Brain Death Laws

The enabling laws leave some leeway for clinicians to define which neurological functions are relevant to the determination of death and to specify how loss of these functions is to be measured. In this context, various medical organizations, including the American Academy of Neurology (14), have formulated detailed guidelines and clinical criteria for determining death by neurological criteria. The laws do require, however, that functions of the "whole" brain—both "higher" cerebral and "lower" brainstem—be taken into account, that the loss of relevant functions be irreversible, and that determinations be made in accordance with prevailing ("ordinary" or "generally accepted") standards of practice. Accordingly, a secure clinical finding of irreversible loss of consciousness will not, by itself, justify a determination of brain death (15). Nor will evidence that all relevant functions are absent justify a diagnosis of death, unless it is also determined that the loss of functions is irreversible. In any event, a determination based on an assessment that omits a step prescribed by relevant practice guidelines, parameters or consensus statements, such as a rigorous apnea test or testing for cough reflexes, could be challenged in court as inconsistent with generally accepted standards of practice (11,16).

Some state laws may impose additional constraints. For example, the Virginia brain death statute requires clinicians to determine specifically with respect to reflexes or functions found to be absent that "further attempts at resuscitation or continued supportive maintenance would not be successful in restoring such (brainstem) reflexes or spontaneous (brain) functions" (7). While this verbiage merely elaborates the requirement of irreversibility of functional loss, a failure to address the issue in the manner contemplated by the statute could be legally problematic.

Aside from constraints that inhere in the definition of brain death and its manner of determination, there are constraints that derive from the fact certain members of the body politic do not either fully understand or fully accept the concept of brain death. Both New Jersey—by statute (8)—and New York—by regulation (13)—direct physicians to make an effort to identify religion-based or other principled objections to use of neurological criteria to determine death. New Jersey would prohibit use of these criteria if a valid objection is asserted by a lawful representative of a putatively "brain-dead" person. New York requires only that a "reasonable accommodation" be made to such an objection. Although physicians in other states may not be subject to such formalized legal strictures, a knowing failure to address or take into account the strongly asserted objections of kinfolk or significant others would raise both legal and ethical concerns. On the legal side, an aggrieved family member might assert a tort claim for intentional infliction or emotional distress if it could be shown that a physician knew or should have known that a family member would be greatly distressed if brain death were declared and precipitously proceeded to make the determination (17). On the ethical side, there is the obligation to behave with sensitivity towards family of a dying or recently deceased patient (18). This would include communicating about the clinical status of a loved one, and bringing the family into deliberations about when to withdraw a ventilator or other "life support."

ERRORS IN DIAGNOSIS OR MANAGEMENT
Concepts of Clinical Error

Clinicians may err in various ways in diagnosing brain death or in handling delicate relationships with families or other legally significant actors. No attempt will be made here to catalogue such errors, many of which will be legally inconsequential. Rather attention will center more generally on the sorts of errors that might be made and on selected court cases that illustrate some of the legal problems that may arise when clinicians determine death by neurological criteria.

Three types of error will be addressed, arbitrarily classified as technical, judgmental and normative. In the area of determining brain death, a technical error is one that results from unintentional or inept misapplication of an assessment measure. Examples might include using a dim light to test pupillary reactions, not obtaining a final arterial Pco_2 determination during an apnea test, or not vigorously enough testing for gag or cough reflexes. A judgmental error is one that results from a failure to conform to generally accepted standards in making a determination of brain death. Examples would be a failure to address a seemingly remote possibility that sedative or other drugs that depress neurological functions might contribute to an individual's unresponsiveness to noxious stimulation, or omitting an apnea test because other clinical evidence of loss of brain functions seems compelling. A normative error derives from a failure to adhere to professional standards of knowledge or behavior. Examples might include lack of knowledge as to the clinical criteria for determining brain death, allowing one's own views about what constitutes death (e.g., that loss of cortical functions equates to brain death) to influence the determination.

Any of these errors could be a potential source of legal difficulties for a clinician. But from a public policy perspective, the greatest concern is the normative error. Such an error implies ignorance, laziness or arrogance. Public perception of these qualities in physicians could severely undermine confidence in their trustworthiness in making the decisions about death that law has delegated to them. Nevertheless, reported legal cases involving challenges to physicians' conduct in making determinations of death by neurological criteria are rare. In these cases, physicians themselves are not the principal targets.

Some Illustrative Cases

The following cases exemplify legal challenges to determinations of brain death. While the involved physicians were not themselves defendants, errors they might have made—whether technical, judgmental or normative—are important considerations in the cases.

People v Eulo

This case (11) established that it is lawful to determine death by neurological criteria in the state of New York. At issue was whether a criminal defendant or the physicians who removed a gunshot victim's mechanical ventilator caused his death. The physicians, including a neurosurgeon, had determined the victim was "brain dead" before the ventilator was removed. A neurologist, testifying as an expert witness for the defendant noted that the apnea test was not rigorously performed and that the electroencephalogram (EEG) which was read as isoelectric had enough artifacts as to cast some doubt on this interpretation. The court nevertheless determined that other evidence of irreversible loss of brain function was sufficient to justify the determination of brain death, and affirmed a jury verdict that the defendant was guilty of murder.

The attending physicians' errors here, if any, were technical. The medical records did not reflect that oxygenation was supplied during the apnea test or that an arterial Pco_2 determination was made, and the physicians had no clear recollection of how the test was performed. While the EEG did not reveal any unequivocal brain wave activity, there were electrical artifacts that could have obscured cerebral rhythms. There was, however, ample evidence that the victim was unresponsive to stimuli, was flaccid and areflexic, was apneic under the test as conducted, and had sustained massive brain injury. Under these circumstances, both trial and appellate courts were willing to accept the conclusion of the attending physicians that the victim was dead by neurological criteria when the ventilator was removed. It should be noted, however, that this case was decided before detailed clinical guidelines concerning brain death had been widely vetted and disseminated. A court today might be less willing to accept a determination resting heavily on an apnea test of uncertain rigor.

In re Alvarado

At issue in this case (16) was the validity of New York's brain deaths regulations (13) as applied to an infant. A clinical determination of brain death was made by attending clinicians within a few hours of the infant's birth and while cardiorespiratory functions were being maintained with a ventilator. When the parents were advised that their baby was brain dead, they insisted that the ventilator not be removed. After further discussion, hospital officials notified the parents that they would remove the ventilator unless forbidden by court order. The mother then initiated legal proceedings to obtain such an order. About 6 weeks after the initial determination of brain death, a court-appointed child neurologist examined the infant. She testified that the baby was immobile, unresponsive to stimuli, had mid-position unreactive pupils, no ocular response to oculocephalic or oculovestibular using ice water caloric testing, no rooting, sucking, cough or corneal reflexes, and did not breathe during an apnea test in which 100% O_2 was delivered via an endotracheal tube. Two electroencephalograms were isoelectric. On cross-examination, the expert conceded that "some brain cells" were "alive" in the medulla—although the basis for this testimony does not appear in the published opinion of the court.

The trial court then concluded that the infant was dead by neurological criteria and that the New York regulations were constitutional as applied in this case. However, it continued a preliminary order restraining the hospital from removing the respirator for an additional 5 days to allow the parents to move the child to another facility or to appeal. The parents appealed and the respirator was continued.

Three months later the state appellate court vacated the trial court decision on the basis of unspecified "new medical findings" indicating that the infant was not brain dead. As part of this ruling, the hospital agreed to seek judicial review before conducting further tests to determine whether the infant was brain dead.

It is most unfortunate that the "new medical findings" were not described in the appellate court's opinion. Based on the expert's admission on cross-examination that some medullary cells were functioning, one can speculate that the infant may have exhibited some response to palatal or tracheal stimulation or that some sort of rudimentary respiratory movements were observed. The error here—if indeed it was an error—could have been technical in the sense of not performing sufficiently vigorous palatal or tracheal stimulation, or judgmental in the sense of not attributing significance to whatever reflex responses might have been observed. Certainly there is no hint of normative error here—unless one takes the position that in the current state of neurological knowledge it is not possible to diagnose brain death in an infant. There was a good faith effort by a knowledgeable physician who applied generally accepted criteria for assessing cerebral and brainstem functions.

People v Lai

In this case (19), a criminal defendant raised the issue of normative error in the determination of brain death. As in the Eulo case (11), the defendant asserted that the physicians who removed a respirator from a "brain-dead" victim caused his death, not the defendant who had shot him in the head. In support of this claim, the defendant secured the testimony of a physician and a priest. Each testified that, under the then current state of technology, death could never be accurately and conclusively diagnosed until after cessation of cardiorespiratory functions. In other words, the physicians allegedly violated a professional normative standard by relying on neurological criteria to diagnose death. The court rejected this argument, citing Eulo for the proposition that it is lawful to determine deaths by neurological criteria when respiratory and circulatory functions are maintained by mechanical means.

Gallups v Cotter

In this case (17), a neurosurgeon and another physician were sued for the tort of outrage. Parents of a brain-injured child alleged that the defendants had failed to obtain parental consent before removing the child's ventilator. The defendants, in consultation with other neurosurgeons, had determined that the child was dead by neurological criteria, having performed several examinations over an 11-day period and having obtained three electroencephalograms, all of which showed no detectable cerebral activity. Testimony at the trial was conflicting as to whether the parents verbally agreed to removal of the ventilator after the determination of brain death was made. The trial judge awarded summary judgment to the defendants because it was found that they had not acted intentionally or recklessly as was required to sustain a claim of outrage under state law. The state supreme court affirmed this ruling, observing that there was no evidence that the defendants "had a desire to inflict extreme emotional distress or that they knew severe emotional distress was likely to result from their actions."

Arguably the defendants made a judgmental error in not assuring themselves that the parents understood their child was dead and were ready emotionally for removal of the ventilator. But neither the trial nor appellate courts viewed this as the sort of error that should produce civil liability, nor was there any suggestion that either court perceived any technical error in the way the physicians made their determination. Since state law authorized determination of death by neurological criteria and the defendants were careful about making their determination, there is no basis for positing a normative error.

In re Haymer

Whether a physician might have erred in determining death or relating to family members was not an issue here (20). However, the court's ruling provides guidance that might forestall a claim of technical or judgmental error in future cases. The court had decided it was lawful to apply neurological criteria to determine death in a 7-month-old child who was being maintained on a mechanical ventilator. It then faced the question of whether the time of death for legal purposes was when brain death was diagnosed or when the ventilator was removed. In choosing the time of diagnosis, the court relied on evidence that there was at that time "irreversible cessation of total brain function, according to usual and customary standards of practice." Most brain death statutes accord with this view so the signal value of the court's ruling is limited. But in states without brain death statutes, this case may be useful to physicians concerned with accurately recording the time of death.

CONCEPTUAL DISAGREEMENT

Nature of the Disagreement

Challenges to the concept of "brain death" can be expressed in theological, philosophical, social/political or medical/scientific terms. Although theological and philosophical arguments undoubtedly influence how law responds to data emerging from medicine and science, these arguments are beyond the scope of this legally oriented chapter. These aspects of the matter can be found in the Presidential Commission report, "Defining Death" (21,22) (see Chapter 9). The emphasis here will be on the role of law in translating whatever medical and social consensus exists about brain death into workable standards and rules.

At the outset, it is clear that there is a substantial, democratically arrived at consensus about the appropriateness of using neurological criteria to determine death. Publicly accountable lawmakers in nearly all states have enacted laws that expressly allow physicians to diagnose death by reference to the functional status of the brain. The decisions of courts in states without such laws have upheld the validity of determinations of brain death when the evidence has shown the accepted clinical criteria were applied. While opponents of brain death laws may contend that the laws were enacted precipitously or ignorantly, there is no apparent popular momentum towards repeal. Nevertheless, it is also clear that there are those who refuse to accept the notion that a person is dead when vital non-neurologic functions can be sustained, sometimes for many months (23) (see Chapters 8 and 9). The disbelief may also be couched as a plea to respect the humanity or religious beliefs of the neurologically impaired, or as skepticism about the reliability of predictions that presently observed unresponsiveness is in fact irreversible.

For those who would undo current state brain death laws, the task is daunting—but hardly inconceivable. State electorates have adopted referenda that override targeted state laws, such as property tax or affirmative action laws, or that create new entitlements that legislators have not chosen to enact, such as access to physician-assisted suicide or to marijuana for medical purposes. More conventionally, citizens can elect representatives who share their views about social issues such as brain death and who can eventually achieve repeal of offending legislation. Concerned citizens can also lobby state officials to sharpen their oversight of decisions to remove ventilators from "brain-dead" patients. Whether such efforts will be mounted or could succeed is highly speculative. But since most regulation of health care decisions occurs at the state and local level, well organized interest groups can concentrate their efforts on elected and appointed officials who are known to them. In a scenario where some states repeal their brain death laws, one could imagine a situation where a person is legally dead in one state but not in another state. In the unlikely event that this occurs, one could imagine that proponents of brain death legislation would respond by lobbying for a federal brain death law that would preempt isolated state laws that bar determination of death by neurological criteria.

Deference to Opposing Views

Widespread repeal of brain death laws seems improbable. But one can still envision modifications in these laws that respond to the beliefs and sensitivities of those who oppose such laws in principle, hold reservations about the scientific foundations of brain death, or who oppose the application of the laws to members of their families. Deference of this sort could take various forms.

One approach is to require by statute or regulation that physicians who propose to determine death by neurological criteria notify patients' next of kin or other lawful representatives prior to making the determination so that those who speak for the patients can raise questions or objections. Both the New Jersey brain death statute (8) and the New York brain death regulations (13) exemplify this approach. The New York regulations do not bar physicians from proceeding to determine death by neurologic criteria once they have heard reservations expressed by patients' representatives, requiring only that physicians make a "reasonable accommodation." The New Jersey statute, however, bars use of neurological criteria to determine death if an attending physician "has reason to believe, on the basis of information provided by a member of the individual's family or any other person knowledgeable about the individual's personal religious beliefs that such a declaration would violate the personal religious beliefs of the individual." This law thus provides for a religion-based veto of the use of neurological criteria to determine death, provided there is evidence that a patient's religious beliefs would be offended by the use of such criteria. The statute does not command physicians to defer to the religious beliefs of family members or to non-religious objections (e.g., that the scientific evidence supporting the reliability of brain death determinations is shaky, that the patient was philosophically opposed to the concept of brain death). But the New Jersey legislature, or any other state legislature, for that matter, could amend state brain death laws to confer a broadly based veto power over the use of neurological criteria to determine death.

Another approach would be to enact laws that impose sanctions on physicians or hospitals for specific sorts of misconduct in determining death by neurological criteria. In light of evidence that many physicians are poorly informed about the concept of brain death and criteria for its determination (24–26), the possibility of an ignorance-based "normative" error is ever present. Accordingly, a law might explicitly penalize physicians who fail to adhere to generally accepted standards and clinical practice parameters in determining death by neurological criteria (e.g., omitting an apnea test, failing to test for sedative drugs in appropriate circumstances), regardless of whether the determination has other legal consequences. Or a law could penalize certain forms of insensitivity in dealing with families or significant others, such as a failure of diligence in trying to locate a family member before determining brain death or failure to advise a family that a patient's condition is such that a brain death determination is being considered.

While relevant case law is sparse, there are a few published opinions that consider what constitutes acceptable conduct in dealing with families or other lawful representatives of neurologically devastated patients when brain death determinations are being made or considered.

In *re Long Island Jewish Medical Center* (27) addresses what constitutes a "reasonable accommodation" under the New York brain death regulations (13). Here parents sued to block a hospital from using neurological criteria to determine the death of their 5-month-old infant, citing their religious beliefs. The suit was filed after the infant's physicians notified the parents they were intending to make such a determination, as was required by the relevant regulations. The hospital's policy manual did not address what "reasonable accommodation" should have been offered. The court then undertook to analyze what steps had actually been taken in order to determine if the requisite accommodation had occurred. It found that the hospital had kept the parents informed of the infant's condition, that its physicians were made available for consultation with the parents, and that the hospital had encouraged the parents to seek a second opinion from an expert of their choosing. After this expert agreed that neurological criteria for death had been satisfied, the hospital then sought a judicial hearing to provide the parents a forum to express their views. The hospital also advised the parents that it was willing to transfer the infant to a facility of the parents' choice. Based on this evidence, the court decided that the hospital had made a "reasonable accommodation" under the regulations, and that the infant was "brain dead with no chance of recovery." It then authorized the hospital to remove the infant's respirator.

It noted its sympathy with the religious convictions of the parents, but interpreted state law as requiring the ruling it made.

Unlike the New Jersey brain death statute (8), the New York regulations do not bar physicians from diagnosing brain death if a religion-based objection is asserted on behalf of a patient. All that is required is a "reasonable accommodation." The Long Island Jewish decision suggests that the essential elements of such an accommodation include providing an opportunity for dialogue and for a second opinion. If a patient's lawful representatives persist in their opposition, a hospital could lawfully remove a respirator if it chose. Alternatively, it could seek a protective judicial order or try to transfer the patient to a facility that is willing to accede to the wishes of the legal representatives. None of these options may be agreeable to a hospital, and it might simply choose to continue use of the respirator on the assumption that cardiac arrest will probably occur within a short time.

In *Dority v Superior Court* (18), parents of a minor child who had been diagnosed as brain dead sought a court order barring removal of the child's mechanical ventilator. After noting that a determination of brain death was lawful under state law, the court commented as follows:

> This does not mean the hospital or the doctors are given the green light to disconnect a life-support device from a brain-dead individual without consultation with the parent or guardian. Parents do not lose all control once their child is determined brain dead. We recognize the parent should have and is accorded the right to be fully informed of the child's condition and the right to participate in a decision of removing the life-support devices. Their participation should pave the way and permit discontinuation of artificial means of life support in circumstances where even those most morally and emotionally committed to the preservation of life will not be offended. Whether we tie this right of consultation to an inherent parental right, the Constitution, logic, or decency, the treating hospital and physicians should allow the parents to participate in this decision.

Thus, even though the state brain death statute did not mandate parental notification prior to a determination of brain death, the court firmly believed that this is something the physicians or hospital should do.

In *Strachan v John F. Kennedy Memorial Hospital* (28), an appellate court upheld parents' tort claim against a hospital based on its delay in releasing the body of their child who had been diagnosed as brain dead after a self-inflicted gunshot wound to the head. The attending physicians had delayed removal of the boy's respirator for 3 days while the hospital administration was obtaining a legal opinion about the lawfulness of the brain death determination and was deliberating about whether to convene a "Prognosis Committee." In characterizing the parental distress that triggered the lawsuit, the court observed as follows:

> The record in this case reveals particularly compelling evidence of distress. Although plaintiffs were told that their son was brain dead and nothing further could be done for him, for three days after requesting that their son be disconnected from the respirator plaintiffs continued to see him lying in bed with tubes in his body, his eyes taped shut, and foam in his mouth. His body remained warm to the touch. Had Jeffrey's body been removed from the respirator when his parents requested, a scene fraught with grief and heartache would have been avoided, and plaintiffs would have been spared additional suffering.

The irony of the ruling in the Strachan case is considerable. In a self-absorbed defensive effort to avoid any liability associated with the determination of death by neurological criteria—at a time when New Jersey had no brain death statute—the hospital incurred liability precisely because of the legalistically driven delay in acting on the clinicians' diagnosis of brain death.

Defendants in several other cases have been more fortunate. In *Smith v Methodist Hospital* (29), an appellate court affirmed a trial court's ruling that the hospital was not guilty of fraud or intentional infliction of emotional distress because of allegedly misleading statements made by a hospital chaplain to parents of a brain-injured child and because of the hospital's alleged failure to advise parents in a timely fashion that physicians believed their child was brain dead. In *Gallups v Cotter* (17), discussed previously, physicians who had allegedly failed to obtain parental consent before removing a ventilator from a brain-dead child avoided liability for the tort of outrage when the court found that they had not acted recklessly or with intent to cause distress to the parents. In *Brown v Delaware Valley Transplant Program* (30), a hospital was sued for mutilation of a corpse, intentional infliction of emotional distress, civil conspiracy and assault for its allegedly wrongful failure to obtain consent to organ donation from relatives of a brain-dead gunshot victim. The court found that the hospital had acted in good faith in relying on the efforts of the state police to locate relatives. Under the Uniform Anatomical Gift Act (31), this sort of "good faith" provided immunity from civil liability for non-consensual harvesting of organs for transplantation.

These escapes from legal accountability notwithstanding, insensitivity to families of brain-dead persons is an invitation to a lawsuit. While hospitals and clinicians may ultimately prevail, financial and other costs of mounting a defense may be considerable. Also, it is difficult to predict how a sympathetic judge or jury might respond to allegations of unfeeling or excessively bureaucratic behaviors on the part of clinicians or hospitals, and regulatory bodies may see fit to impose fines or accreditation-related sanctions for such behavior.

REDEFINING BRAIN DEATH: A SLIPPERY SLOPE?

Pitfalls of a Qualitative Definition of Life

Current law adopts a quantitative approach to defining death. Clinicians are enjoined to determine whether relevant neurological or cardiorespiratory functions are present or absent. With respect to the brain, they are not asked to characterize the quality of life of a person whose essential brain functions are lacking. Although consciousness may be preeminent among these essential functions, a finding that consciousness is irreversibly lost will not by itself, under applicable law, justify a diagnosis of brain death (2,6,15,32). Evidence that brainstem functions are absent is also required. The assessment of these functions largely consists of determining whether certain reflexes (e.g., pupillary, corneal, oculocephalic, oculovestibular, gag, cough) or respiratory drive are present or absent. To some, the insistence that death not be declared until all brainstem reflexes are undetectable betrays a failure to appreciate that human life, or the life of the person, is over when consciousness is lost (33). In the Cruzan case (32), where the Supreme Court ruled that the state of Missouri could require parents of an adult daughter in a persistent vegetative state (PVS) to prove by "clear and convincing" evidence that she would not want her life sustained by a feeding tube before allowing removal of the tube, Justice Stevens observed in his dissenting opinion:

> The Court . . . permits the State's abstract, undifferentiated interest in the preservation of life to overwhelm the best interests of Nancy Beth Cruzan, interests which would . . . be served by allowing her guardians to exercise her constitutional right to discontinue medical treatment . . . The meaning of her life should be controlled by persons who have her best interests at heart—not by a state legislature concerned only with the preservation of human life . . . However commendable may be the State's interest in human life, it cannot pursue that interest by appropriating Nancy Cruzan's life as a symbol for its own purposes . . .

In other words, some individuals may believe that it is in their best interests to die when consciousness is irreversibly lost. Extrapolating to the determination of brain death, a state should arguably not inflict its brainstem-oriented concept of death on persons who clearly believe that life is over when consciousness is gone.

Some legal scholars have endorsed the notion that human death occurs when that part of the brain that determines consciousness—wherever that locus is—is lost (34,35). Their arguments assume neurological findings that consciousness is both lacking and will never return are reliable enough to eliminate a significant risk that life-support will be withdrawn from a person who might potentially regain consciousness. The risk of error is small if generally accepted criteria are applied and the latest technical advances, such as functional neuroimaging, are utilized (36). But it may not be small enough to convince legislatures or courts to enlarge the definition of death to include irreversible loss of consciousness alone.

If laws were changed to equate death with loss of consciousness, concerns would likely arise over the possibility that the definition of "unconsciousness" might gradually be expanded to include the barely or minimally conscious, and then the severely retarded, the severely demented, and the severely psychotic. In such persons, the nature and content of consciousness may not be ascertainable by even skilled observers and examiners. It might then be concluded that they are, although undeniably responsive to nonverbal—and perhaps some verbal—stimuli, permanently lacking in the sort of human consciousness that affords autonomy or "quality" in their lives. It would be far-fetched to suggest that they would thereupon be treated as "brain dead" and no longer deserving of respect or compassion. But allowing qualitative measures a place in assessments of whether "life" is present evokes concerns of this nature.

Line-Drawing and the Courts

In several cases addressing decisions about ending life in persons with severe neurological impairment, courts have tried to balance the state's interest in protecting life of its citizens and the individual's interest in bringing an intolerable life to an end. In so doing, courts have not only drawn a line between brain death and permanent unconsciousness, they have also tried to clarify what conditions of severe neurological impairment will justify decisions to end life. These judicial efforts may be instructive in evaluating concerns about slippery slopes.

In the seminal *Quinlan* case (15), the New Jersey Supreme Court explicitly distinguished PVS from brain death and recognized that it was being asked to approve a decision—removal of a ventilator—that could lead to the death of a young woman in a PVS. The court ultimately concluded that the removal would be lawful if the evidence was "clear and convincing" that this would be her choice if she were capable of exercising it. Although proof was skimpy as to what her preference might be, the court viewed her loss of cognitive function as the sort of predicament that would justify a person's choosing to discontinue life support. Accordingly, it authorized her father to exercise a "substituted judgment" on her behalf to remove the respirator. In short, even though Ms. Quinlan was not dead, her life in a PVS was bad enough that she had a right to bring that severely compromised life to an end. In response to arguments that removal of the ventilator would constitute homicide, the court asserted that the legal cause of her death would be her underlying neurological condition, not the act of removal, and that her constitutional right of self-determination outranked any state interest in protecting her life. Thus, although she was not dead by neurological criteria, her condition was such that she (through her family) could rationally opt for death.

The *Conroy* case (37), which arose in New Jersey not long after *Quinlan,* posed the question of whether a family member of a minimally conscious elder with severe and permanent neurological impairments could direct removal of her feeding tube. As in *Quinlan,* brain-death was not at issue and there was little compelling evidence as to her actual preferences. She died before the court finally ruled in her case. Nevertheless, the court formulated a three-pronged test to be applied in future cases of this nature. The third prong would permit removal of life support when a person's preferences are unknown and where it is shown, by objective criteria, that removal is in a person's "best interests." This determination is made by weighing the benefits of continued life against its burdens. The court viewed intractable pain as the relevant burden for purpose of this calculus, thus seemingly excluding an individual's emotional distress over his or her condition as a factor to be weighed.

Over a stinging dissent that it was endorsing suicide and euthanasia, Massachusetts' high court ruled in the *Brophy* case (38) that removal of a feeding tube from a vegetative patient was lawful where there was evidence that, during sapient life, he had indicated he would not want to survive in such a state. The dissenter, Justice Nolan, wrote as follows:

> Paul Brophy will die as a direct result of the cessation of feeding . . . He will not die from the aneurysm which precipitated loss of consciousness, the surgery which was performed, the brain damage that followed on the insertion of the G-tube. He will die as a direct result of the refusal to feed him.

The majority of the court concluded, however, that protecting Brophy's right to choose not to survive in a state of permanent unconsciousness trumped any societal interest in prolonging his life.

The issue of whether ending life support for a permanently unconscious patient is homicide was raised directly in the *Barber* case (39). Attending physicians were charged with murder for acts—removal of a respirator and feeding tube—that they knew would cause the death of patient who was comatose following a complication of elective surgery. In ordering dismissal of the murder charge, a California appellate court conceded that the physicians' actions were intentional and resulted in death. But it also concluded that in this particular circumstance, the physicians had no legally enforceable duty to sustain life.

In the context of potential organ transplantation, the Florida Supreme Court recently declined to hold that an anencephalic infant is brain-dead (40). The child's respiration was being supported by a mechanical ventilator, and her parents wanted to donate her organs for transplantation while they were still viable. But since the Florida brain death statute requires proof that all functions of the brain are absent before brain-death is declared, the court denied the parents' request. This decision harmonizes with the Uniform Anatomical Gift Act which requires that heart-beating organ donors be brain dead before their organs can be removed (31).

The United States Supreme Court waded into the debate with its ruling in the *Cruzan* case. At issue was whether the state of Missouri could require, before permitting removal of a feeding tube from a young woman in a PVS, "clear and convincing" evidence that removal accorded with preferences she had expressed while conscious. The Court held that the state's interest in protecting life was a constitutional justification for such a requirement. But it also assumed that Ms. Cruzan had a constitutionally protected right to refuse a feeding tube if that was shown to be her choice. When her parents eventually produced "clear and convincing" evidence that removal of the tube was what she would have wanted, the Missouri courts allowed removal.

In his concurring opinion in *Cruzan,* Justice Scalia criticized the majority of the Court for undertaking to balance the interests of individuals against those of the state. In his view, it is a legislative or political decision as to how far a state can go in protecting the lives of its citizens. Thus, if the democratically elected legislature of a state chooses to bar or criminalize removals of life support from living patients, it can constitutionally do so. Consonant with this view is the Court's recent ruling that the constitution does not bar states from criminalizing physician-assisted suicide (41,42). A seeming corollary is that a state could also enact laws that explicitly authorize removals of life support from permanently unconscious patients, or even laws that redefine death to include permanent loss of consciousness.

Legislative Redefinition of Death

Under current law, death can be determined only on the basis of irreversible loss of cardiorespiratory or whole-brain functions. But judicial tolerance of decisions to remove life support from vegetative patients, highlighted in the previous section, raises the possibility that legislatures might entertain proposals to revise the standards for determining death to include irreversible loss of consciousness (so-called "neocortical death"). Proponents might choose to emphasize that consciousness is the defining feature of human personhood, that the interests of the state in sustaining vegetative life—as determined by the courts—is minimal, that the burdens on families and society of prolonged survival of vegetative patients are substantial, and that it is ultimately futile to expend societal and personal resources on persons who cannot benefit from this. Arguments of this sort have probably helped persuade courts to approve removals of life support from vegetative patients under certain circumstances and have probably encouraged wider use of advance directives by those who cannot endure the thought of being maintained indefinitely in a vegetative state.

Challenges to a legislative expansion of the concept of brain death are readily envisioned. One is that consciousness is too elusive a concept on which to base a determination of death. It is one thing to assert that absence of detectable responses to external stimuli indicates destruction of those areas of the brain necessary for integrated functioning as a human being. But it is quite a different matter to assert that a person who is apparently awake, moves, breathes without a respirator, has roving eye movements, grimaces, and utters sounds is as dead as one who is flaccid, immobile, and requires a ventilator and pharmaceutical support to maintain homeostasis. A second challenge would be some version of a slippery slope argument. For example, if death is redefined to include permanent loss of consciousness, what about the minimally or barely conscious? Their prognosis is probably no better than that of a person who meets diagnostic criteria for PVS. Are they to be regarded as dead too? What of other neurologically devastated subjects who are totally dependent for survival on large allocations of societal resources? A third sort of challenge is more philosophical or abstract. A focus on cognition as the touchstone of human personhood risks devaluing of lives of those who fail to meet a majoritarian norm of intelligence. Thus, the law should endeavor to protect all humans, not simply one of its preferred attributes (i.e., cognition).

Assuming that legislatures could be persuaded by medical or scientific experts that permanent unconsciousness can be reliably diagnosed, they would have at least two options. One is to redraft the brain death statutes so as to allow death determined on the basis of a permanent loss of cerebral (or neocortical) functions, or permanent loss of consciousness, provided determinations are made in accordance with generally accepted standards of medical practice. A second option would be to provide legal immunity for clinicians who choose to remove or withhold life support from patients who are diagnosed as having a permanent loss of cerebral functions or of consciousness. To achieve this sort of legislation would require compelling evidence that permanent loss of cerebral functions or consciousness is diagnosable with a high degree of medical certainty. Whether available data are sufficiently compelling is certainly contestable (23,43). Prospects for an expanded legislative definition of brain death are, therefore, seemingly remote. Clinicians engaged in making decisions about removals of life support from neurologically impaired patients who do not meet existing criteria of brain death will not, for the foreseeable future, be able to rely on brain death laws to immunize themselves from legal inquiry. Fortunately for them, evolving case law provides considerable legal cover for decisions that rest on careful neurological assessments and that can be fairly interpreted as implementing patients' preferences (35).

CONCLUSION

By statute or judicial ruling, all states in the United States empower clinicians to employ neurological criteria to determine death. The criteria must be ones that are generally accepted by the medical profession, patients' medical records should clearly reflect that the criteria have been applied and met, and any special requirements of state laws should be satisfied (e.g., reasonable accommodation to religion-based concerns of family members). If these conditions exist, the risk of legal entanglements from applying neurological criteria to determine death is minimal. Problems may arise, however, if clinicians fail to inform themselves about the specifics of relevant state laws, or fail to appreciate the needs of families for adequate information, explanation or emotional support. And clinicians should remain mindful that laws permitting use of neurological criteria to determine death do not apply to decisions regarding removal of ventilators or feeding tubes from persons diagnosed as permanently unconscious but whose brainstem functions are wholly or partially intact. Although courts may allow removal of life support from these unconscious persons, the legal justification is not that they are already dead (44–47).

APPENDIX: LEGAL BASIS FOR DETERMINING DEATH BY NEUROLOGICAL CRITERIA IN THE UNITED STATES

State	Primary legal authority
Alabama	ALA. CODE sec. 22-31-1 to 4 (1997)
Alaska	ALASKA STAT sec. 09.65.120 (Michie 1998)
Arizona	State v Fierro, 603 P. 2d 74 (AZ 1979)
Arkansas	ARK. CODE ANN. secs. 20-17-101 (Michie 1991)
California	CAL. HEALTH & SAFETY CODE, secs 7180-7183 (West 1998)
Colorado	COLO. REV. STAT. SECS. 12-36-136 (West 1998)
Connecticut	CONN. GEN. STAT. ANN. SEC. 19a-278(b),(c) (West 1997)
Delaware	DEL. CODE. ANN., tit.24, sec. 1760 (1997)
District of Columbia	D.C. CODE ANN. SEC. 6-2401 (1981)
Florida	FLA. STAT. ANN. sec. 382.009 (West 1997)
Georgia	GA. CODE ANN. SEC. 31-10-16 (1996)
Hawaii	HAW REV. STAT. sec. 327C-1 (1993 & Supp. 1997)
Idaho	IDAHO CODE sec. 54-1819 (1994a & Supp. 1998)
Illinois	ILL. COMP. STAT. ANN. 755/50-2 (West 1993)
Indiana	IND. CODE ANN. sec. 1-1-4-3 (Michie 1998)
Iowa	IOWA CODE ANN. sec. 702.8 (West 1993)
Kansas	KAN. STAT. ANN. sec. 77-205 (1997)

Kentucky	KY. REV. STAT. ANN. sec. 446-400 (Michie 1985 & 1996)
Louisiana	LA. REV. STAT. ANN. sec 9:111 (West 1991)
Maine	ME. REV. STAT. ANN. tit. 22, secs. 2811-2813 (West 1997)
Maryland	MD. HEALTH-GEN I CODE ANN. secs. 5-201,202 (1997)
Massachusetts	Commonwealth v Golston, 366 NE 2d 744 (MA 1977)
Michigan	MICH. COMP. LAW ANN. secs. 333.1021,1024 (West 1992)
Minnesota	MINN. STAT. ANN. sec. 145.135 (West 1998)
Mississippi	MISS. CODE ANN. sec. 41-36-3 (1993 & Supp. 1998)
Missouri	MO. ANN. STAT. sec. 194.005 (West 1996 & Supp. 1998)
Montana	MONT. CODE ANN. sec. 50-22-101 (1997)
Nebraska	NEB. REV. STAT. ANN. secs. 71-7201 to 71-7203 (Michie 1996)
Nevada	NEV. REV. STAT. ANN. sec. 451.007 (Michie 1997)
New Hampshire	N.H. REV. STAT. ANN. sec. 141D:1,2 (1996)
New Jersey	N.J. REV. STAT. sec. 26.6A-1 to 8 (1996)
New Mexico	N.M. STAT. ANN. sec. 12-2-4 (Michie 1978)
New York	People v Eulo, 472 NE 2d 286 (NY 1984)
North Carolina	N.C. GEN. STAT. sec. 90-323 (1997)
North Dakota	N.D. CENT. CODE sec. 23-06.3.01 to .3-02 (1991)
Ohio	OHIO REV. CODE ANN. sec. 2108.30 (West 1993)
Oklahoma	OKLA. STAT. ANN. tit. 63, secs. 3121-3123 (West 1997)
Oregon	OR. REV. STAT. sec. 432.300 (1997)
Pennsylvania	PA. STAT. ANN. tit.35, secs. 10,201-10,203 (West 1993)
Rhode Island	R.I. GEN. LAWS sec. 23-4-16 (1996)
South Carolina	S.C. CODE ANN. sec. 44-43-450, -460 (Law Co-op 1985 & 1997)
South Dakota	S.D. CODIFIED LAWS sec. 34-25-18.1 (Michie 1994)
Tennessee	TENN. CODE ANN. sec 68.3-501 (1996)
Texas	TEX. HEALTH & SAFETY CODE ANN. sec. 671.001 (West 1992)
Utah	UTAH CODE ANN. secs. 26-34-1 to -2 (1998)
Vermont	VT. STAT. ANN. tit.18, sec. 5218 (Michie 1982)
Virginia	VA. CODE ANN. sec. 54.1-2972 (Michie 1998)
Washington	In re Bowman, 617 P. 2d 731 (WN 1980)
West Virginia	W.VA. CODE, sec. 16-10-1 to -4 (1997)
Wisconsin	WIS. STAT. ANN. sec. 146.71 (West 1997)
Wyoming	WYO. STAT. ANN. sec. 35-29-202 to -103 (Michie 1997)

REFERENCES

1. *In re Bowman,* 617 P 2d 731 (WN 1980).
2. Uniform Determination of Death Act, *12 Uniform Laws Annotated* 589 (West 1993 and West Supp 1997).
3. Weyrauch S. Acceptance of whole-brain criteria for determination of death: a comparative analysis of the United States and Japan. *UCLA Pacific Basin Law J* 1999;17:91–123.
4. ALA CODE sec 23-31-1 to 4 (1997).

5. W VA CODE sec 16-10-1 to -4 (1997).
6. Uniform Brain Death Act, *12 Uniform Laws Annotated* 65 (1978).
7. VA STAT sec 54-1-2972 (1997).
8. NJ STAT ANN 26-6A-5 (1987, suppl 1994).
9. *State v Fierro,* 124 Ariz 182, 603 P 2d 74 (1979).
10. *Commonwealth v Golston,* 373 Mass 249, 366 NE 2d 744 (1997), cert den 98 S Ct 777 (1978).
11. *People v Eulo,* 63 NY 2d 341, 472 NE 2d 286 (1984).
12. *State v Guess,* 244 Conn 761, 715 A 2d 643 (1998).
13. NY COMP CODES, RULES 7 REGS, Title 10, sec 400.16(d),(c)(3) (1992).
14. Quality Standards Subcommittee of the American Academy of Neurology. Practice parameters for determining brain death in adults. *Neurology* 1995;45:1012–1014.
15. *In re Quinlan,* 355 A 2d 647 (NJ 1976), *cert den sub nom Garger v NJ,* 429 US 922 (1976).
16. *In re Alvarado,* 547 NYS 2d 190 (S Ct NY Cty 1989), vacated 550 NYS 2d 353 (S Ct App Div 1990).
17. *Gallups v Cotter,* 544 So 2d 585 (AL 1988).
18. *Dority v Superior Court,* 193 Cal Rptr 288 (CA App 4th Dist 1983).
19. *People v Lai,* 516 NYS 2d 300 (S Ct App Div 1987).
20. *In re Haymer,* 115 Ill App 3d 349, 450 NE 2d 940 (IL App 1983).
21. President's Commission for the Study of Ethical Problems in Medicine and Biomedical and Behavioral Research. *Defining death: a report on the medical, legal and ethical issues in the determination of death.* Washington, DC: U.S. Government Printing Office, 1981.
22. Beresford HR. Review of Defining Death. *NY Law School Law Rev* 1982:27:1273–1280.
23. Shewmon DA. Chronic "brain death" conceptual consequences. *Neurology* 1998;51:1538–1545.
24. Mejia RE, Pollack MM. Variability in brain death determination practices in children. *JAMA* 1995; 274:550–553.
25. Youngner SJ, Landesfeld S, Coulton CJ, et al. "Brain death" and organ retrieval. *JAMA* 1989; 261:2205–2210.
26. Youngner SJ. Defining death: a superficial and fragile consensus. *Arch Neurol* 1992;49:570–572.
27. *In re Long Island Jewish Medical Center,* 641 NYS 2d 989 (S Ct Queens Cty 1996).
28. *Strachan v John F. Kennedy Memorial Hospital,* 109 NJ 523, 538 A 2d 346 (1988).
29. *Smith v Methodist Hospital,* 569 NE 2d 743 (IN Ct App 1991).
30. *Brown v Delaware Valley Transplant Program,* 420 Pa Super 84, 615 A 2d 1379 (1992).
31. Uniform Anatomical Gift Act, *8 Uniform Laws Annotated* 15 (1973).
32. *Cruzan v Director,* 497 US 261 (1990).
33. Veatch RM. *Death, dying and the biological revolution: our last quest for responsibility.* New Haven: Yale University Press, 1989, 16–35.
34. Smith DR. Legal recognition of neocortical death. *Cornell Law Rev* 1986;71:850–888.
35. Stacy T. Death, privacy and the free exercise of religion. *Cornell Law Rev* 1992;77:490–595.
36. Multi-Society Task Force. Medical aspects of the persistent vegetative state. *N Engl J Med* 1994; 330:1499–1508,1572–1579.
37. *In re Conroy,* 486 A 2d 1209 (NJ 1985).
38. *Brophy v New England Sinai Hospital,* 398 Mass 417, 497 NE 2d 332 (1986).
39. *Barber v Superior Court,* 147 Cal App 1006, 195 Cal Rptr 414 (1983).
40. *In re T.A.C.P.,* 609 So 2d 588 (FL 1992).
41. *Vacco v Quill,* 117 S Ct 2293 (1997).
42. *Washington v Glucksberg,* 117 S Ct 2258 (1997).
43. Childs NL, Mercer WN. Late improvement in consciousness after post-traumatic vegetative state. *N Engl J Med* 1996;334:24–25.
44. Beresford HR. Legal aspects of termination of treatment decisions. *Neurol Clin* 1989;7:775–787.
45. MacDonald AC. Organ donation: the time has come to refocus the ethical spotlight. *Stanford Law Policy Rev* 1997;8:177–184.
46. Stern MD. "And you shall choose life"—futility and the religious duty to preserve life. *Seton Hall Law Rev* 1995;25:997–1014.
47. Strasser M. The futility of futility? On life, death, and reasoned public policy. *Maryland Law Rev* 1998;57:505–557.

9

Philosophical and Ethical Aspects of Brain Death

James L. Bernat

Neurology Section, Dartmouth-Hitchcock Medical Center, Lebanon, New Hampshire

The idea that irreversible absence of brain function was the equivalent of death began in the 12th century with the writings of the famous Jewish physician and philosopher Moses Maimonides. Maimonides noticed that decapitated humans exhibited muscular twitches for a short time immediately following decapitation. He asserted that decapitated humans were dead instantly and that such muscle movements were not a sign of life because they lacked the central direction that was indicative of the soul (1).

"Brain death" is a colloquial term meaning human death determined by showing the irreversible cessation of clinical brain functions. Although "brain death" is a term hallowed by decades of consensual medical and legal usage, it remains an unfortunate term. The term is misleading because it may falsely suggest that there are two types of death: brain death and ordinary death, rather than reflecting the reality that there is only one type of death that can be measured in two ways. Moreover, the term may falsely suggest that it is only the brain and not the human being that is dead. This misunderstanding of the term "brain death" itself may be responsible for much of the public and professional confusion about this concept. Because the term "brain death" has become a permanent fixture of our vocabulary, those using it should take care to use it precisely to prevent any further ambiguity. (Most recently, the expression "brain dead" even has entered the American slang vernacular to refer derogatorily to a dull-witted person.)

The idea that a human being who has suffered irreversible loss of clinical brain functions is dead—irrespective of the presence of mechanically-supplied ventilation and supported circulation—has become accepted throughout most of the Western world over the past three decades (2–4). Interestingly, public acceptance of this concept began before there existed a rigorous philosophical argument showing that the brain dead patient was truly dead. In 1981, the President's Commission for the Study of Ethical Problems in Medicine and Biomedical and Behavioral Research published Defining Death as their first project (5).

Thereafter, the President's Commission's panel of medical experts and numerous medical societies and other organizations published guidelines for physicians on the determination of death using brain death tests (6–10). These test batteries are essentially alike, requiring the irreversible absence of all clinical brain functions as proved by the presence of complete unresponsivity, apnea, and brainstem areflexia, the absence of significant potentially reversible metabolic or toxic conditions, and the presence of a structural brain lesion sufficient to account for the clinical findings. Over the past decade, there has been a current trend for additional countries to accept brain death, including some countries that had previously rejected the concept, such as Denmark and Japan. In this chapter, the philosophical concepts underlying the acceptance of brain death in public policy will be discussed, and will highlight areas of current controversy.

THE PHILOSOPHICAL BASIS FOR REGARDING BRAIN DEATH AS HUMAN DEATH

The intuitive appeal of the concept of brain death led to its general acceptance as a standard of death by the Western public throughout the late 1960's and 1970's. By the time of the President's Commission report in 1981, most American states already had enacted statutes of death incorporating brain death. Yet even in the decade prior to 1981, several scholars worked to provide a theoretical foundation for brain death based upon the indispensable role of the brain in the phenomenon of human death. Interestingly, the Harvard Ad Hoc Committee report did not base its "new criterion of death" on any conceptual basis. Rather, the report cited two pragmatic justifications: to permit termination of medical treatment in hopeless cases and to permit vital organ procurement (3).

In 1972, Alexander Capron and Leon Kass wrote an influential article proposing a model brain death statute (11). In defense of their model statute, they argued that agreeing upon a conceptual model of death was a necessary precondition before physicians could develop tests for death. In the same year, the Institute of Society, Ethics, and the Life Sciences (known now as the Hastings Center) published a task force report emphasizing the distinction between the concept and criteria of death, and outlining the ideal characteristics of death criteria (12). In 1976, Robert Veatch, one of the authors of the Hastings Center task force report, published a book-length analysis of his version of the concept and criteria of death, which will be discussed later (13). In 1977, Frank Veith and colleagues published an influential two-part article in *JAMA* showing the conceptual validity of brain death and arguing that brain death determination is consistent with Judeo-Christian religious traditions (14,15).

In a conference of the New York Academy of Sciences in 1978 on brain death, the conference chairman, Julius Korein, emphasized the distinction between constructs, concepts, and criteria of death, and presented a conceptual basis for brain death based upon the theoretical biology of critical systems (16). Korein argued that the brain is the single "critical vital system" whose irreversible destruction was both a necessary and sufficient condition for death. When the critical system of an organism was destroyed, the organism as an individual, coherent, functioning entity no longer existed. The human organism whose critical system has been destroyed inevitably increases entropy and inexorably progresses to states of greater disorder. Korein has further expanded this theme in his more recent writings (17).

In 1981, Charles Culver, Bernard Gert, and James Bernat published the first of two articles attempting to establish the conceptual validity of whole-brain death as a formulation of death (18,19). This analysis has been refined further in three additional articles over the past two decades (20–22). This analysis was cited in the President's Commission report *Defining Death* as the philosophical basis of the whole-brain formulation of death (5). Several subsequent writings on the definition of death have continued the debate. Noteworthy works include those of David Lamb (23) and Karen Gervais (24). Two recently published conference proceedings edited by Calixto Machado (25) and Stuart Youngner and colleagues have generated interest as well (26).

Scholars who accept a brain death paradigm for human death generally fall into one of three categories known as: whole-brain, higher brain, and brainstem formulations of death (21). The whole-brain theorists believe that the irreversible loss of all clinical functions of the cerebral hemispheres and brainstem is sufficient for death. By contrast, the higher brain theorists hold that only loss of hemispheric functions is sufficient for death, while the brainstem advocates hold that loss of all brainstem functions alone is sufficient for death. The brainstem concept is accepted in the United Kingdom. In all other jurisdictions in the world that accept brain death, including the United States, the whole-brain concept is codified. A small group of scholars, but no jurisdictions anywhere in the world, endorse the higher brain formulation of death.

An Analysis of Death

Why, in the second half of the 20th century, has there been a heated argument about the determination of human death? The explanation can be found by analyzing the profound impact of medical technology. Prior to the mid-20th century, death was a unitary phenomenon: when one vital system ceased, such as the brain, heartbeat, or breathing, all the others quickly and inevitably ceased. It was not necessary to consider whether a human organism was dead when only certain vital systems ceased because such cases were impossible. Thus, the absence of heartbeat, breathing, and consciousness served as utterly reliable signs of death.

With the advent of the mechanical ventilator, however, it became possible to support respiration (and thereby maintain circulation) despite the complete destruction of the brain. But now the life status of patients with destroyed brains and mechanically supported respiration became ambiguous. Such so-called "brain dead" patients shared some features of alive patients: heartbeat, circulation, digestion, and excretion of urine, for example. But they also shared some features of dead patients: unresponsiveness to all stimuli, absence of movement, and apnea. Now, physicians alone no longer were able to determine whether such patients were alive or dead because the traditional determination of death had become ambiguous as a result of technology. First it was necessary to rigorously define death to enable physicians to decide which clinical signs to measure to determine death.

We have argued that a rigorous analysis of the meaning of human death in our current technological age could be accomplished best by conducting four sequential tasks: determining the assumptions, definition, criterion, and tests of death (18,22). Determining the assumptions is a philosophical task that frames the overall paradigm in which the concept of death is understood. Identifying the definition of death is a philosophical task that requires making explicit the indispensable characteristic of death implicit in our consensually agreed upon concept of death. Choosing a general criterion showing that the definition has been fulfilled by being both necessary and sufficient for death is both a philosophical and medical task. Finally, choosing a set of tests and procedures to show that the criterion has been satisfied is purely a medical task.

Assumptions About Death

A prerequisite for any rigorous analysis of death is to agree on a set of assumptions about the nature of death (18,22). Although it is true that not all scholars share these assumptions, it is difficult to imagine ever achieving consensus on a philosophical analysis of death unless these are accepted because the assumptions frame the argument by defining the paradigm. For example, the failure to agree with the assumption that death is fundamentally a biological phenomenon creates a paradigm noncongruence that precludes choosing a definition of death. Similarly the failure to agree that all organisms must be either alive or dead makes it impossible to choose a unitary criterion of death.

Assumption 1

"Death" is a nontechnical word that we use correctly. The goal of any analysis of the concept of death is to make explicit the implicit consensually-accepted meaning of the word "death," not to contrive a redefinition to satisfy a social, political, philosophical, or medical agenda. In this analysis the purview is restricted to the death of the human organism, not the death of a human cell, tissue or organ. As will be shown, brain death is the most explicit rendering of the concept of human death.

Assumption 2

Death is a biological phenomenon. We all agree that the practices surrounding dying, death determination, burial, and mourning have rich and profound social, cultural, anthropological, legal, religious, and historical aspects. But fundamentally, death, like life, is a biological phenomenon. It is a term that we all use correctly to refer to the cessation of the life of a living organism. It is a term that applies only to living organisms or tissues, unless one uses it metaphorically, such as with the phrase "the death of a culture." All living organisms must die and only living organisms may die. As a biological phenomenon, death is not arbitrarily contrived by society but is an independent and immutable physical point terminating the life of an organism.

Assumption 3

Death is irreversible. It is not possible to return from being dead. Irreversibility is not merely a limitation of current technology; it is an intrinsic and inescapable element of the definition of death. Patients recovering after resuscitation from cardiac arrest have recovered from dying, not death. Similarly, patients later describing so-called "near-death" experiences may have returned from dying but not from being dead.

Assumption 4

Death is an event and not a process. Alive and dead are the only two possible underlying states of any organism. All organisms must be either alive or dead; they cannot be neither nor both. Conversely, dying and bodily disintegration are processes that happen to organisms: dying while the organism is alive, and disintegration after the organism is dead. Death is the event that separates the processes of dying and disintegration. Death must be an event because the transition from the bodily state of alive to that of dead is inherently discontinuous and sudden because there is no intervening state.

Assumption 5

Death should be able to be determined by physicians with a high degree of reproducibility and accuracy, at least in retrospect, using relatively simple bedside tests. The tests for death should be delineated and validated to eliminate the possibility of false-positive determinations.

The Definition of Death

The philosophical task of identifying the essential and indispensable characteristic defining death requires a rigorous explication of the biological phenomenon of death. Because death no longer is a unitary event, we can no longer rely on the simultaneous cessation of functioning of all vital organs. Certain definitions are not plausible. For example, defining death as the cessation of all bodily cellular functions is not what we mean by death because hair and nails continue to grow for several days after the usual declaration of death, and because cell lines may be kept alive for months or years in cell culture. Similarly, defining death as the time the soul leaves the body may represent a belief about death shared by many but is not what even religious individuals mean by death.

I define death as the permanent cessation of the critical functions of the organism as a whole (22). The organism as a whole is an old concept in theoretical biology that refers to the unity and functional integrity of an organism, not to the mere sum of the parts of an organism (27). The concept of organism as a whole emphasizes how the parts of an organism interact with each other to comprise an integrated, unified, working whole. Functions of the organism as a whole are stratified on a level higher than functions of organs or tissues because they serve the overall health and unity of the organism. Critical functions are those without which the organism as a whole cannot function.

Critical functions of the organism as a whole include the vital functions of respiration and circulation, a set of integrating, regulating, and homeostatic functions that are crucial for life, and consciousness, which is necessary for obtaining hydration, nutrition, protection, and numerous other activities that serve the organism's continued health. The complete and irreversible loss of these critical functions represents the death of the organism because it is no longer functioning as a whole. It is not possible for organ subsystems to continue to function when the organism as a whole ceased functioning except with technological support, such as that which has become available during the past 40 years. The brain-dead patient whose circulation is maintained due to support from mechanical ventilation and vasopressor and anti-diuretic agents represents such an example.

The Criterion of Death

What criterion best satisfies this definition? The criterion that is both necessary and sufficient for death is the irreversible cessation of the clinical functions of the whole brain. A review of the physiology of the critical functions of the organism as a whole reveals that they are subserved within the brainstem, hypothalamus, thalamus, and cerebral hemispheres. Respiration and blood pressure control are generated in the brainstem. The complex array of regulatory, feedback, and homeostatic mechanisms are integrated in the brainstem and hypothalamus. Consciousness requires the ascending reticular activating system of the brainstem, thalamus, and cerebral hemispheres. Therefore, the clinical functions of each major part of the brain must be absent for the cessation of the critical functions of the organism as a whole. This concept has been called the "whole-brain" formulation of death.

The term "clinical functions" refers to observable functions that can be tested at the bedside. The pupillary reflexes to light and dark are examples of clinical functions. These reflexes require integrated neural circuits with an afferent limb, efferent limb, and central processing. They function to maximize vision in varying degrees of ambient light and serve the organism as a whole. They can be tested easily and reproducibly at the bedside with great accuracy. The term "clinical functions" does not extend, however, to the physiological functioning of individual cells that may be measured using laboratory techniques. Thus the concept of the irreversible loss of all clinical functions of the brain does not necessarily require the permanent cessation of function of every cell in the brain; only that the coordinated clinical product of such functioning is lost. Thus, some rudimentary EEG activity may be recordable despite brain death (28).

The only major function of the organism as a whole not directly located in the brain is heartbeat. The heart has its own pacemaker and can continue to beat as long as the blood is oxygenated and other physiologic conditions are maintained. The brainstem does exert some degree of control over heartbeat rate and strength, and circulation through the sympathetic and parasympathetic innervation of the heart and the medullary control of blood pressure. But, as brain dead patients show, heartbeat in some instances can continue for substantial periods of time if other bodily physiologic functions are maintained through technological means.

Beginning in the 1970's, several scholars argued that brainstem and hypothalamic functions were not crucial to the concept of brain death, and only the loss of consciousness and cognition by damage to the cerebral hemispheres and thalamus was necessary for death (29–31). This position, known as the higher brain formulation, asserted that death was defined as "the irreversible loss of that which is considered to be essentially significant to the nature of man" (29). The criterion satisfying this definition was the irreversible cessation of consciousness and cognition. Because damage to the thalamus or cerebral hemispheres alone could create such a state, patients in persistent vegetative states (PVS) and neonates with anencephaly presumably would be declared dead according to the higher brain formulation.

The higher brain formulation creates several problems as a concept of death (22). First, it violates assumption #1 by being a contrived redefinition of death, because it classifies patients as dead who are universally regarded as alive, such as those in a PVS. Second, it applies only to *Homo sapiens*, whereas a coherent biological concept of death should apply equally well to other higher animals, and third, it creates a slippery slope problem because it does not make clear how much brain damage is necessary for death. The higher brain formulation fails as a model of death because it does not map out to our consensual concept of death. Its proper place is not in a definition of death but in determining criteria to discontinue life-sustaining therapy on a hopelessly brain-damaged patient.

The criterion of death accepted in the United Kingdom is the irreversible cessation of functions of the brainstem. From a practical perspective, so-called "brainstem death" is quite similar to whole-brain death in that the clinical sets of tests to determine death are identical. As Christopher Pallis has correctly pointed out, even whole-brain death tests focus primarily on showing cessation of brainstem function (32). This accurate observation reflects the course of events occurring during the pathophysiology of brain death.

Brain death is produced most commonly by massive traumatic brain injury, diffuse hypoxic-ischemic damage, and massive intracranial hemorrhage. These primary insults create markedly elevated intracranial pressure, which at some time in nearly every case, exceeds mean arterial blood pressure. Intracranial circulation then ceases and, as a result, neurons not already put to an end by the primary insult die by the secondary ischemic insult. The profound intracranial hypertension produces syndromes of intracranial brain herniation and the ultimate absence of brainstem function confirms the conclusion and irreversibility of this process and represents the valid sign of whole-brain death.

The concept of brainstem death, however, permits death to be determined in those very unusual but well-recorded cases, predominantly pontine, hemorrhage in which there is a brainstem catastrophe that spares the thalami and cerebral hemispheres (33,34). Cerebral circulation usually is preserved in such cases. Although it is difficult to imagine how awareness could be preserved given destruction of the brainstem ascending reticular activating system—despite the intact thalami and cerebral hemi-spheres—the theoretical possibility of a profound locked-in syndrome with preserved awareness cannot be excluded confidently merely on the basis of a neurologic exam-ination. This outside chance is one reason why the concept of brainstem death is not as coherent as whole-brain death as a formulation of human death (see Chapter 4).

The Tests of Death

The determination of death is a clinical procedure performed at the bedside. This fact remains true when death is determined using brain death tests. There are two sets of clinical tests to determine death that reflect the two fundamental clinical circum-stances of critical care: in the presence of or in the absence of mechanical ventilation. For the patient in whom mechanical ventilation is neither in use nor planned, the pro-longed absence of heartbeat and breathing represent valid signs of death because they inevitably lead to complete hypoxic-ischemic destruction of the brain. Of course, the patient is not dead until the brain has been totally infarcted because the patient could be resuscitated prior to that point and retain some preserved neurologic function; hence the organism would remain alive.

The exact duration required for the absence of heartbeat and breathing to unequiv-ocally determine death is not known. This question has been studied most recently in conjunction with attempts to stipulate the duration of asystole necessary to determine the moment of death for the non–heart-beating organ donor (35). In this context, the Institute of Medicine stipulated 5 min of asystole as the point at which death could be determined using cardiopulmonary tests (36). This point represented an increase from the 2-min asystole standard employed in the original Pittsburgh protocol that was based on theory but little empirical data (37). The Institute of Medicine argued that after 5 min of asystole, the patient would not auto-resuscitate. Further, because artificial resuscitation would not be attempted, the patient was dead. However, it is clear that while such a patient is incipiently dying, the patient is not unequivocally dead until many minutes later, at which time the brain has totally infarcted from hy-poxic-ischemic damage (38,39).

For the patient who is mechanically ventilated, specific brain death tests must be used, as detailed in Chapter 4. These tests show permanent cessation of the clinical functions of the whole brain. They have been validated extensively and have been ac-cepted widely.

OPPONENTS TO THE CONCEPT OF BRAIN DEATH

There have been opponents to the concept of brain death since it was first intro-duced in the 1960's. The higher brain advocates have been among the most long-standing critics. But they did not oppose the idea of brain death, they merely wished to change its criterion from the whole brain to the cerebral hemispheres and thalamus. Despite a quarter century of writings, however, the higher brain theorists have not succeeded in convincing any jurisdiction in the world to change its brain death laws from the whole brain to the higher brain formulation.

During the 1990's, a new group of brain death opponents emerged to refute the overall concept of brain death. The current opponents argue three positions: (a) brain death is philosophically incoherent as a concept of human death; (b) brain death is a legal fiction that no longer serves a useful social purpose; and (c) brain death is incompatible with the belief systems of Christianity and Judaism.

Conceptual Confusion and Legal Fiction

Within the past decade, several scholars have pointed out purported inconsistencies in the whole-brain formulation. Robert Veatch, the most persistent critic, argued that the principal claim allegedly made by whole brain advocates was false, namely that all functions of the entire brain were absent, because some brain dead patients retained rudimentary EEG activity and antidiuretic hormone secretion (40,41). This theme also was echoed by Baruch Brody and Amir Halevy (42). These scholars cited the Uniform Determination of Death Act, the model death statute proposed by the President's Commission codifying the whole-brain formulation, which states in part: "an individual who has sustained . . . irreversible cessation of all functions of the entire brain, including the brainstem, is dead" (5). Notwithstanding the sweeping language of the Uniform Determination of Death Act, the discussion in the President's Commission report preceding the statute makes perfectly clear that the word "functions" applies only to clinical functions as I have defined them, not to laboratory-measured cellular physiologic activities. Thus, the whole-brain formulation remains compatible with any degree of preserved neuronal activity that does not contribute to a clinical function.

In a prominent article, Robert Truog argued that brain death is an anachronism that should be abandoned (43). He pointed out that when the brain death concept was formulated over 30 years ago, there was no acceptable professional standard to discontinue ventilators and other forms of life-sustaining therapy on hopelessly ill patients with massive brain damage. By declaring the patient dead, these life-sustaining measures could be legally discontinued. But now that there are standards available to permit withholding or withdrawal of life-sustaining therapy, we no longer need to rely on brain death. The one remaining use of brain death is to permit unpaired vital organ donation. Truog then suggested that unpaired vital organ donation could be accomplished through means other than by declaring the donor brain-dead, such as by relying on patient or family consent in a hopelessly ill, dying patient beyond harm.

In a similar vein, Robert Taylor believes that brain death represents a "legal fiction" that is no longer necessary in contemporary society (44). He pointed out that the concept of brain death is similar to the legal fiction of "legal blindness." We all know that many patients determined to be legally blind are not in fact completely blind. But they have visual loss so severe that for legal purposes their visual loss is functionally equivalent to blindness. The concept of legal blindness is a useful fiction created by law that permits these patients to receive society's benefits that are reserved for the blind. Similarly, he argues, we all know that brain dead patients are not really dead; we just employ this convenient legal fiction to permit unilateral termination of life-sustaining treatment and multiorgan procurement.

It is certainly true that brain death no longer is a necessary condition for discontinuing life-sustaining therapy and that its major utilitarian benefit is to permit unpaired vital organ transplantation and unilateral termination of therapy. However, the fact that it may be useful today in only these ways does not necessarily alter the coherence of whole brain death as a concept of death. In contrast to these criticisms, those of Alan Shewmon that brain death is conceptually incoherent are more serious challenges.

Chronic Cases and Spinal Integration

In a series of scholarly articles, Alan Shewmon has produced the most serious challenges thus far to the brain death concept (45–47). These articles are particularly fascinating because prior to 1994, Shewmon was one of the strongest advocates of brain death (45). Like Robert Taylor and the philosopher Josef Siefert (48), Shewmon now holds that the human is not dead until circulation ceases irreversibly. In the circulation formulation that he proposes, the brain is simply one organ among many and enjoys no special significance in death determination.

Shewmon cites two lines of data to support his contention. First, he criticizes the whole-brain concept's reliance on the brain's unique capacity to integrate, regulate, and maintain homeostasis. He points out that other structures in the body, especially the spinal cord, perform integrating functions, and that therefore it is arbitrary to impart special value to those particular integrating and regulating functions performed by the brain. Thus, even accepting death as the permanent cessation of the critical functions of the organism as a whole, he argues that loss of whole brain function does not necessarily achieve this standard.

Shewmon's second line of argument features cases he classifies as "chronic brain death." He recently reported a series of patients who had been declared brain dead but who had respiration and other functions supported technologically for prolonged periods of months, and in one remarkable case, for years (47). Several of these patients were pregnant women who were physiologically maintained for several months to permit live birth of viable neonates by Cesarean delivery. Shewmon argues that it is counterintuitive to the concept of death to consider that dead people could do what those brain dead have done, such as gestate infants, grow (as in the case of the child maintained for years), or have circulation and other organ functions maintained for prolonged periods.

In response to the integration/regulation criticism, one may point out that these capacities of the brain are not the sole evidence of functions of the organism as a whole. As noted earlier, the vital functions of respiration and circulation as well as consciousness are critical functions. In response to the chronic cases, I would first respectfully question whether all the patients Shewmon cited were unequivocally brain dead. Some of the cases were not reported in sufficient detail to be certain that they had undergone proper tests for apnea, for example. Granted, however, that many of these patients were unequivocally brain dead, I view the existence of the "chronic" cases as rare outliers that reveal evidence that our intensive care technology now occasionally succeeds in producing instances of physiological support of heroic proportions. But it cannot be concluded that the existence of these cases necessarily must change our concept of death.

Religious Opposition

Despite the early claim by Veith and colleagues that brain death is compatible with the traditional beliefs of Christianity and Judaism (14), a number of authorities have opposed brain death on religious grounds since the introduction of the concept. For example, Paul Byrne and colleagues have claimed for over 20 years that the purported equivalence between death and the loss of brain functions is incompatible with traditional Christian beliefs about the unity of the soul and body (49,50).

In Judaism, disagreement also exists about brain death. One prominent Orthodox rabbi, David Bleich, argues that brain death is incompatible with the ancient body of Jewish law, the halacha (51). Another leading Orthodox rabbi, Moshe Tendler, claims that whole-brain death is consistent with halachic law because it produces the equivalent of physiological decapitation, which clearly is death (52). There remains an active debate by rabbinic authorities on this important question, but brain death determination has been banned by at least some Orthodox Jewish rabbis who insist upon continued treatment of the brain dead patient (53).

The Roman Catholic church has accepted brain death in the past (54,55) and permits multiorgan procurement and transplantation at Catholic hospitals around the world. Pope Pius XII stated in the 1950's that death determination was the domain of physicians and not of the church. Now, however, given the philosophical basis of brain death as a concept of death, the Vatican Pontifical Academy for Life recommended formally adopting brain death as a doctrine of the church magisterium. This position was approved by Pope John Paul II in August, 2000.

Until recently, Islam rejected brain death but the council of Islamic Jurisprudence Academy in 1986 supported the concept of brain death in the kingdom of Saudi Arabia and other Islamic countries. The acceptance of organ donation by various religious groups is discussed in greater detail in Chapter 7.

ETHICAL ISSUES

A number of challenging ethical issues arise during the determination of brain death and the care of the brain-dead patient. Many of these issues result from ignorance or confusion by the public or professionals about the concept of brain death (56). Other issues emanate from the unique physiology of the brain dead patient, in which certain bodily systems continue functioning despite death. Several public policy issues have been created as our pluralistic society attempts to incorporate this biophilosophical concept into workable public laws. Like most ethical issues, there are plausible arguments supporting both sides of the question.

Family Opposition to Brain Death

Most experienced neurologists, neurosurgeons, and intensivists have encountered the unpleasant and awkward situation in which family members of a brain dead patient insist that the patient's "life-sustaining" treatment be continued because of their hope for recovery. In defense of their position, family members may cite stories of people about whom they have heard, who made dramatic and unexpected recoveries from coma, proving wrong their physicians who had issued emphatically hopeless prognoses. Despite careful and compassionate explanations by the physician about the nature of brain death, some family members continue to insist that all treatments be continued (57,58). How should the physician respond to such requests?

The compassionate physician should attempt to explain the difference between coma and brain death, that the patient is dead, and that any attempts at further treatment are therefore futile. The physician should investigate to learn if there is a religious or cultural basis to the family member's nonacceptance of brain death (see Chapter 7). If this is present, as for example in the case of some devout Orthodox Jews, the physician should respect the religious belief and continue treatment pending inevitable asystole. In recognition of this situation, in 1991, New Jersey became the first state to enact a law providing citizens with a religious exemption from brain death determination (59).

More often, however, the reason for nonacceptance of brain death is emotional: the unwillingness of the family member to accept the finality of the patient's tragic death. In these cases, further counseling is advisable by the physician, nurse, chaplain, or social worker. Often, continued treatment for a day or two is sufficient to convince the skeptical family member that further support is hopeless, permitting them to accept the inevitability of death. There is not a legal duty to continue treatment temporarily in these cases but the approach represents the most compassionate course of action.

MATERNAL BRAIN DEATH AND SPERM DONATION

There have been a number of well-reported tragic cases of maternal brain death during pregnancy, usually the result of traumatic brain injury or intracranial hemorrhage. In several of these cases, the father of the fetus or other family member has requested that physiologic support of the dead mother be continued until the fetus was mature enough to permit live birth (60–62a). In a few of these cases, physiologic support of the mother has been successful for as long as four months and live, healthy babies have been born by Cesarean delivery (60). Surely these cases demonstrate the technological virtuosity of heroic intensive care unit physicians vicariously, successfully managing the complex physiologic disorders of the brain dead patient, but they also raise challenging ethical questions. Should continued physiologic support of the dead mother be conducted insofar as it violates her dignity and interrupts the closure of her life? Who should decide upon further treatment? What is the authority of physicians to recommend or discourage such an act?

Some commentators have argued that the physician has an ethical responsibility to encourage live births in these cases, based on the dual ethical duties of the obstetrician to the mother and the fetus. When the mother's life no longer can be saved, then the duty to rescue is transferred to the fetus (61,62). This duty increases with increasing fetal maturity because of the increased chance of successful rescue. There is general agreement, at least in the setting of marriage, that the father is best poised to consent for such treatment of the prospective mother. Only the father of the child can adequately weigh the various risks and benefits of continued treatment, including the emotional and financial costs of hospitalization, single parenthood, harm to the mother, and neonatal abnormality.

In men, there have been recent reports of obtaining viable sperm from brain-dead men by seminal vesicle massage electroejaculation (63). Similarly, viable sperm have been harvested from men after ordinary cardiopulmonary death by postmortem surgical orchidectomy followed by cryopreservation. These cases raise many of the same difficult ethical questions as do the cases of brain dead pregnant women.

Education and Research on Brain Dead Patients

Ethical questions arise when brain dead patients are considered as subjects for teaching or research purposes. Newly deceased patients, including the brain dead, have been used as teaching subjects for decades. The practice of using brain dead patients for teaching purposes raises the obvious ethical question of whether informed consent had been obtained (64). Yet obtaining consent is fraught with difficulty because it entails asking the relatives of a recently deceased patient the ghoulish question of permission for doctors to manipulate the loved one's corpse for practice. Proponents claim that there is less harm to the patient and family by practicing without first seeking consent.

Although there is no clear answer to this question, there is probably no reason why this particular clinical instance should obviate the ordinary ethical requirement of obtaining informed consent. The solution proposed by Orlowski and colleagues of implied consent in the absence of a prior refusal (65) is not satisfactory unless people universally were aware of this practice and given ample opportunity to refuse.

Similarly, there have been several published research studies using brain dead patients as human subjects, particularly for protocols that are so dangerous that they could not be performed safely on living subjects (66,67). For many research studies, the brain dead patient represents an ideal research subject: numerous bodily systems remain intact, such as circulation and the immune system, but the patient cannot possibly be harmed by the protocol because he is already dead. Yet, this practice again raises ghoulish issues of consent that must be obtained carefully and compassionately.

John La Puma outlined the following criteria for performing research on brain dead subjects (68). The diagnosis of brain death should be unequivocal. The experiment should be approved by the appropriate institutional review board. The experiment should be important and one likely to yield valuable information that could not be obtained in any other way. The experiment should be limited to minutes or hours.

Informed consent of the appropriate proxy decisionmaker must be obtained. The human subject's dignity should not be violated by the experiment, and any additional charges for the patient's medical and hospital care resulting from the research should be borne by the investigators.

Personal Choice of Death Criteria

One outstanding public policy question is the extent to which our pluralistic society and democratic process should permit individual discretion in the choice of death criteria. The answer to this question turns fundamentally on our accepted paradigm of death. For those who believe that the moment of death primarily is a social construct defined solely by customs and laws, and is not a fixed point of biological reality, there can be tremendous variation among societies and individuals (69–71). Yet for those, such as I, who hold that death is primarily a biological phenomenon, but one for which we construct pragmatic social policies on the basis of their social acceptance, there can be less variation.

Robert Veatch suggests that legal death statutes should provide "conscience clauses" enabling patients to choose in advance whether they wish to be declared dead using whole-brain, higher brain, or cardiovascular criteria (69). Steven Miles supports this view stating that our laws "could offer individuals a choice from a menu of socially acceptable definitions of death" (71). I am skeptical about both the conceptual basis of this idea and the practical consequences of it. Conceptually it abuses biology by making the determination of death a purely social matter. Practically, I can foresee chaos at the bedside of the dying patient as physicians try to figure out what definition of death the patient or family wish to employ. I see further confusion in attempting to implement such a policy in a society that already is confused about brain death.

The Dead Donor Rule in Multiorgan Transplantation

Although it is beyond the scope of this chapter to consider the many ethical issues introduced by multiorgan procurement and transplantation, I conclude with a brief discussion of one topic related to the brain-dead donor, that of the dead donor rule. The dead donor rule has been the ethical axiomatic foundation of the program of vital multiorgan transplantation since the practice was begun in the 1960's. This rule holds that the multiorgan donor must first be dead before unpaired vital organs can be procured. Its corollary is that it is wrong to kill living patients for their organs no matter how ill the patients are or how much good for others can be accomplished by doing so. To a large extent, I believe that the public acceptance of our current practice of multiorgan procurement is the result of public confidence that living patients cannot and will not be used as multiorgan donors.

Several scholars recently have advocated that we change or abandon the dead donor rule (72). For example, Robert Truog believes that we no longer need this rule to continue our successful multiorgan transplantation program. He argues that we can use dying patients who are "beyond harm" with their informed consent, or that of their family (43). The controversy surrounding the use of anencephalic infants as multiorgan donors also featured several scholars advocating for modifying the dead donor rule to permit living anencephalic neonates to serve as multiorgan donors (73,74). Even the American Medical Association Council on Ethical and Judicial Affairs recently advocated permitting multiorgan procurement from not yet dead anencephalic infants until an outcry of protest from members and other medical societies forced them to reverse their position (75).

I believe that the democratic traditions of our pluralistic society should permit a large degree of personal freedom in our decisions to choose to continue or to terminate our own life-sustaining therapy. However, this freedom should not extend to choosing a definition of death. The definition of death remains a biological entity. The social issue of personal choice is the question of when to terminate life-sustaining therapy. This question can and should be best answered without changing the definition of death.

I also fear that eliminating the dead donor rule will lead to a reduction in public confidence about our multiorgan transplantation program because prospective donors may fear that physicians will wish them to die sooner to procure their organs. Similarly, the benefits from using anencephalic infants as organ donors does not justify the harm to society resulting from sacrificing the dead donor rule (76,77).

REFERENCES

1. Pernick MS. Back from the grave: recurring controversies over defining and diagnosing death in history. In: Zaner RM, ed. *Death: beyond whole-brain criteria.* Dordrecht, Netherlands: Kluwer Academic Publishers, 1988:17–74.
2. Mollaret P, Goulon M. *Le coma dépassé (mémoire préliminaire). Rev Neurol* 1959;101:3–15.
3. A definition of irreversible coma: report of the Ad Hoc Committee of the Harvard Medical School to Examine the Definition of Brain Death. *JAMA* 1968;205:337–340.
4. Pernick MS. Brain death in a cultural context: the reconstruction of death 1967–1981. In: Youngner SJ, Arnold RM, Schapiro R, eds. *The definition of death: contemporary controversies.* Baltimore: Johns Hopkins University Press, 1999:3–33.
5. President's Commission for the Study of Ethical Problems in Medicine and Biomedical and Behavioral Research. *Defining death: medical, legal and ethical issues in the determination of death.* Washington, DC: U.S. Government Printing Office, 1981.
6. Wijdicks EFM. Determining brain death in adults. *Neurology* 1995;45:1003–1011.
7. Practice parameters for determining brain death in adults (summary statement): report of the Quality Standards Subcommittee of the American Academy of Neurology. *Neurology* 1995;45:1012–1014.
8. Criteria for the diagnosis of brain stem death: review by a working group convened by the Royal College of Physicians and endorsed by the Conference of Medical Royal Colleges and Their Faculties in the United Kingdom. *J R Coll Physicians Lond* 1995;29:381–382.
9. Canadian Neurocritical Care Group. Guidelines for the diagnosis of brain death. *Can J Neurol Sci* 1999;26:64–66.
10. Guidelines for the determination of death: report of the Medical Consultants on the Diagnosis of Death to the President's Commission for the Study of Ethical Problems in Medicine and Biomedical and Behavioral Research. *Neurology* 1982;32:395–399.
11. Capron AM, Kass LR. A statutory definition of the standards for determining human death: an appraisal and a proposal. *Univ Penn Law Rev* 1978;121:87–118.
12. Refinements in criteria for the determination of death: an appraisal. A report by the Task Force on Death and Dying of the Institute of Society, Ethics, and the Life Sciences. *JAMA* 1972;221:48–53.
13. Veatch RM. *Death, dying, and the biological revolution: our last quest for responsibility.* New Haven: Yale University Press, 1976:21–54.

14. Veith FJ, Fein JM, Tendler MD, et al. Brain death. I. A status report of medical and ethical considerations. *JAMA* 1977;238:1651–1655.
15. Veith FJ, Fein JM, Tendler MD, et al. Brain death. II. A status report of legal considerations. *JAMA* 1977;238:1744–1748.
16. Korein J. The problem of brain death: development and history. *Ann N Y Acad Sci* 1978;315:19–38.
17. Korein J. Ontogenesis of the brain in the human organism: definitions of life and death of the human being and person. *Adv Bioethics* 1997;2:1–74.
18. Bernat JL, Culver CM, Gert B. On the definition and criterion of death. *Ann Intern Med* 1981; 94:389–394.
19. Bernat JL, Culver CM, Gert B. Defining death in theory and practice. *Hastings Cent Rep* 1982; 12:5–9.
20. Bernat JL. The definition, criterion, and statute of death. *Semin Neurol* 1984;4:45–52.
21. Bernat JL. How much of the brain must die in brain death? *J Clin Ethics* 1992;3:21–26.
22. Bernat JL. A defense of the whole-brain concept of death. *Hastings Cent Rep* 1998;28:14–23.
23. Lamb D. *Death, brain death and ethics.* Albany: State University of New York Press, 1985.
24. Gervais KG. *Redefining death.* New Haven: Yale University Press, 1986.
25. Machado C, ed. *Brain death: proceedings of the Second International Conference on Brain Death. Developments in Neurology V.* Amsterdam: Elsevier Science, 1996.
26. Youngner SJ, Arnold RM, Schapiro R, eds. *The definition of death: contemporary controversies.* Baltimore: Johns Hopkins University Press, 1999.
27. Loeb J. *The organism as a whole.* New York: G. P. Putnam's Sons, 1916.
28. Grigg MM, Kelly MA, Celesia GG, et al. Electroencephalographic activity after brain death. *Arch Neurol* 1987;44:948–954.
29. Veatch RM. The whole-brain–oriented concept of death: an outmoded philosophical formulation. *J Thanatol* 1975;3:13–30.
30. Green MB, Wikler D. Brain death and personal identity. *Philos Public Affairs* 1980;9:105–133.
31. Youngner SJ, Bartlett ET. Human death and high technology: the failure of the whole-brain formulation. *Ann Intern Med* 1983;99:252–258.
32. Pallis C. Further thoughts on brain stem death. *Anaesth Intensive Care* 1995;22:20–23.
33. Ogata J, Imakita M, Yutani C, et al. Primary brainstem death: a clinico-pathological study. *J Neurol Neurosurg Psychiatry* 1988;51:646–650.
34. Kosteljanetz M, Øthrstrøm, Skjødt S, et al. Clinical brain death with preserved cerebral circulation. *Arch Neurol Scand* 1988;78:418–421.
35. Youngner SJ, Arnold RM. Ethical, psychosocial, and public policy implications of procuring organs from non–heart-beating cadaver donors. *JAMA* 1993;269:2769–2774.
36. National Academy of Sciences Institute of Medicine. *Non–heart-beating organ transplantation: medical and ethical issues in procurement.* Washington, DC: National Academy Press, 1997.
37. University of Pittsburgh Medical Center. Management of terminally ill patients who may become organ donors after death: the University of Pittsburgh Medical Center policy and procedure manual. *Kennedy Inst Ethics J* 1993;3:A1–A15.
38. Lynn J. Are patients who become organ donors under the Pittsburgh protocol for non–heart-beating donors really dead? *Kennedy Inst Ethics J* 1993;3:167–178.
39. Menikoff J. Doubts about death: the silence of the Institute of Medicine. *J Law Med Ethics* 1998; 26:157–165.
40. Veatch RM. The impending collapse of the whole-brain definition of death. *Hastings Cent Rep* 1993; 23:18–24.
41. Veatch RM. Brain death and slippery slopes. *J Clin Ethics* 1992;3:181–187.
42. Halevy A, Brody B. Brain death: reconciling definitions, criteria, and tests. *Ann Intern Med* 1993; 119:519–525.
43. Truog RD. Is it time to abandon brain death? *Hastings Cent Rep* 1997;27:29–37.
44. Taylor RM. Re-examining the definition and criterion of death. *Semin Neurol* 1997; 17:265–270.
45. Shewmon DA. Recovery from "brain death": a neurologist's apologia. *Linacre Q* 1997;64:30–96.
46. Shewmon DA. "Brainstem death," "brain death," and death: a critical re-evaluation of the purported equivalence. *Issues Law Med* 1998;14:125–145.
47. Shewmon DA. Chronic "brain death": meta-analysis and conceptual consequences. *Neurology* 1998; 51:1538–1545.
48. Seifert J. Is "brain death" actually death? *Monist* 1993;76:175–202.
49. Byrne PA, O'Reilly S, Quay PM. Brain death—an opposing viewpoint. *JAMA* 1979;242:1985–1990.
50. Evers JC, Byrne PA. Brain death—still a controversy. *Pharos* 1990;53:10–12.

51. Bleich JD. Establishing criteria of death. In: Rosner F, Bleich JD, eds. *Jewish bioethics.* New York: Sanhedrin Press, 1979:277–295.
52. Tendler MD. Cessation of brain function: ethical implications in terminal care and organ transplants. *Ann N Y Acad Sci* 1978;315:394–397.
53. Rosner F. The definition of death in Jewish law. In: Youngner SJ, Arnold RM, Schapiro R, eds. *The definition of death: contemporary controversies.* Baltimore: Johns Hopkins University Press, 1999:210–221.
54. Pontifical Academy of Sciences. *Working Group on the Determination of Brain Death and Its Relationship to Human Death.* Vatican City: Scripta Varia 83, 1992.
55. Pontifical Council for Pastoral Assistance. *Charter for Health Care Workers.* Boston: St. Paul Books and Media, 1994.
56. Youngner SJ, Landefeld CS, Coulton CJ, et al. "Brain death" and organ retrieval: a cross-sectional survey of knowledge and concepts among health professionals. *JAMA* 1989;261:2205–2210.
57. Miedema F. Medical treatment after brain death: a case report and ethical analysis. *J Clin Ethics* 1991; 2:50–52.
58. Hardwig J. Treating the brain dead for the benefit of the family. *J Clin Ethics* 1991;2:53–56.
59. Olick RS. Brain death, religious freedom, and public policy: New Jersey's landmark legislative initiative. *Kennedy Inst Ethics J* 1991;4:275–288.
60. Bernstein IM, Watson M, Simmons GM, et al. Maternal brain death and prolonged fetal survival. *Obstet Gynecol* 1989;74:434–437.
61. Loewy EH. The pregnant brain dead and the fetus: must we always try to wrest life from death? *Am J Obstet Gynecol* 1987;157:1097–1101.
62. Kantor JE, Hoskins IA. Brain death in pregnant women. *J Clin Ethics* 1993;4:308–314.
62a. Feldman DM, Borgida AF, Rodis JF, et al. Irreversible brain injury during pregnancy: a case report and review of the literature. *Obstet Gynecol Surv* 2000;55:708–714.
63. Swinn M, Emberton M, Ralph D, Smith M, Serhal P. Retrieving semen from a dead patient. *BMJ* 1998;317:1583–1585.
64. Burns JP, Reardon FE, Truog RD. Using newly deceased patients to teach resuscitation procedures. *N Engl J Med* 1994;331:1652–1655.
65. Orlowski JP, Kanoti GA, Mehlman MJ. The ethics of using newly dead patients for teaching and practicing intubation techniques. *N Engl J Med* 1988;319:439–441.
66. Coller BS, Scudder LE, Berger HJ, et al. Inhibition of human platelet function *in vivo* with a monoclonal antibody: with observations on the newly dead as experimental subjects. *Ann Intern Med* 1988; 109:635–638.
67. Nelkin D, Andrews L. Do the dead have interests? Policy issues for research after life. *Am J Law Med* 1998;24:261–291.
68. La Puma J. Discovery and disquiet: research on the brain-dead. *Ann Intern Med* 1988;109:606–608.
69. Veatch RM. The conscience clause. How much individual choice in defining death can our society tolerate? In: Youngner SJ, Arnold RM, Schapiro R, eds. *The definition of death: contemporary controversies.* Baltimore: Johns Hopkins University Press, 1999:137–160.
70. Brock DW. The role of the public in public policy on the definition of death. In: Youngner SJ, Arnold RM, Schapiro R, eds. *The definition of death: contemporary controversies.* Baltimore: Johns Hopkins University Press, 1999:293–307.
71. Miles S. Death in a technological and pluralistic culture. In: Youngner SJ, Arnold RM, Schapiro R, eds. *The definition of death: contemporary controversies.* Baltimore: Johns Hopkins University Press, 1999:293–307.
72. Arnold RM, Youngner SJ. The dead donor rule: should we stretch it, bend it, or abandon it? *Kennedy Inst Ethics J* 1993;3:263–78.
73. Diaz JH. The anencephalic organ donor: a challenge to existing moral and statutory laws. *Crit Care Med* 1993;21:1781–1786.
74. Walters JW. Yes—the law on anencephalic infants as organ sources should be changed. *J Pediatr* 1989;115:825–828.
75. Council on Ethical and Judicial Affairs, American Medical Association. The use of anencephalic neonates as organ donors. *JAMA* 1995;273:1614–1618.
76. Committee on Bioethics, American Academy of Pediatrics. Infants with anencephaly as organ sources: ethical considerations. *Pediatrics* 1992;89:1116–1119.
77. Steinberg A, Katz E, Sprung CL. The use of anencephalic infants as organ donors. *Crit Care Med* 1993;21:1787–1790.

10

Organ Procurement and Preparation for Transplantation

Steve F. Emery* and Kerri M. Robertson[†]

*LifeSource, Upper Midwest OPO, Inc., Rochester, Minnesota, and [†]Department of
Anesthesiology, Duke University Medical Center, Durham, North Carolina

After all is said and done, the challenge turns to obtaining consent for organ donation
and protecting the vital organs until their recovery for grafting. Today, organ transplants are increasingly common surgical procedures, supported by 90% of the public
(1,2). Due to advances in transplant surgery techniques and immunosuppressive
medications, increasingly more patients with end stage organ failure can be treated
with a transplant. Since the availability of cyclosporine, survival rates have improved
dramatically and organs other than kidneys have been transplanted.

The number of recipients placed on the waiting list for organs far exceeds the number of organs recovered for transplant and this trend continues (1). The prime limit-
ing factor for increasing the number of organs available for transplantation is obtaining consent from brain-dead patients' next-of-kin. According to recent surveys, there
is a disappointing actual consent rate for organ donation of less than 50% (1,3–5).
Several factors have been identified that may increase the consent rate and include
education of health care professionals and the public, but also federal and state legislation (6,7). These factors, along with improved medical management of brain-dead
patients, may increase the number of organs available for transplantation but skepticism remains. Recommended standard ways to approach a family are extrapolated
from surveys, retrospective studies, opinion, and rationalization, as hard data are not
available. A serious effort should be undertaken to prospectively study the tools to
improve organ donation. This chapter presents insights into the administration of
transplantation, offers a guide for conversations with the family, and a template for
medical management and recovery process of the donor.

ADMINISTRATION OF ORGAN PROCUREMENT

Prior to 1987, the system of allocating organs in the U.S.A. was haphazard at best.
A national system was not in place to list patients, collect data on organ donors and
transplant recipients, or ensure the equitable distribution of organs. The National
Transplant Act of 1984 developed the current oversight system of the Organ Procurement and Transplant Network (OPTN) (8).

The United Network for Organ Sharing (UNOS; www.unos.org) was awarded the
OPTN contract by the federal government in 1987. Every hospital that performs or-

gan transplants must be certified by UNOS and abide by its rules and policies to receive organs for transplantation. Likewise, every Organ Procurement Organization (OPO) that recovers organs for transplantation must be certified by the Health Care Financing Authority (HCFA). The goals of UNOS, as stated in its Articles of Incorporation are to:

1. Establish a National Organ Procurement and Transplantation Network under the Public Health Services Act;
2. Improve the effectiveness of the nation's renal and extrarenal organ procurement, distribution, and transplantation systems by increasing the availability of, and access to, donor organs for patients with end-stage organ failure;
3. Develop, implement, and maintain quality assurance activities; and
4. Systematically gather and analyze data and regularly publish the results of the national experience in organ procurement and preservation, tissue typing, and clinical organ transplantation (9).

The UNOS board of directors is comprised of transplant surgeons, OPO representatives, donor family members, transplant recipients, and other interested individuals or organizations. The board sets national organ allocation policy and minimal listing criteria for potential transplant recipients. All patients awaiting organ transplantation, as well as all organ donors, must be registered with UNOS which operates the Organ Center. The Organ Center assists with the placement of organs and registration of potential recipients on the waiting list.

While UNOS oversees all organ donations, OPOs work directly with the organ donors. Most OPOs are independent, private, not-for-profit organizations whose sole function is to work with all aspects of organ donation. Some OPOs continue to be part of individual transplant centers. HCFA assigns OPOs a specific geographic area of operation and certifies them every two years based on the number of organ donors and organs recovered for transplantation per million population (10). Currently there are 63 OPOs that cover the United States and Puerto Rico (www.transweb.org). Independent OPOs are governed by a board of directors that is comprised of transplant surgeons from each transplant center in its service area, a neurosurgeon or neurologist, a histocompatibility representative, and members of the public. All OPOs are funded by HCFA and transplant centers who receive organs recovered by the OPO. OPOs bill a standard acquisition charge (SAC) to the receiving transplant center for every organ transplanted. The SAC (in simplified terms) calculates the cost per organ by adding up all expenses incurred to recover each organ and dividing by the number of organs transplanted. Services provided by OPOs generally include: 24-h availability, immediate response to organ donor referrals, organ donor case management, public and professional education, and donor family aftercare. OPO coordinators generally have a background as a nurse, physician assistant, or paramedic. They receive training on all aspects of organ donation including family approach, donor management, organ allocation policy, and operating room recovery procedures (11). After one year of experience, OPO coordinators are eligible to take the certified procurement transplant coordinator board examination to demonstrate competency measured by national standards (12).

In some modified form, procurement organizations are in place in countries outside the United States. Organ donation programs range from those that are well established and active (e.g., Europe) to programs that are in their infancy (e.g., Japan). Laws concerning organ donation and brain death vary drastically worldwide. Some countries (Austria, Sweden, and Spain) have so-called presumed (implied) consent to organ donation. Others require informed consent (United States, Germany, the Netherlands).

Spain (www.msc.es/ont/ing) has long been a recognized worldwide leader in organ donation with approximately 31 organ donors per million population annually. These rates (82%) are twice as high as other European countries and higher than the United States, with an estimated 24 organ donors per million. Spain's utilization of coordinators who are either specially trained physicians or nurses and presumed consent laws may explain their superb consent rate (13).

EuroTransplant (www.eurotransplant.nl), which includes the countries of Austria, Belgium, Germany, the Netherlands, and Luxembourg, is one of the oldest transplant consortiums in the world (Table 10-1). Other well established programs include France Transplant; Scandiatransplant (Denmark, Finland, Iceland, Norway, and Sweden); and the United Kingdom Transplant service (United Kingdom and Ireland). Like Japan, most other Asian countries are only beginning to develop transplantation programs with brain-dead organ donors instead of living donors and non-heart-beating cadaveric donors. Through 1996, only Hong Kong, Malaysia, The Philippines, Singapore, Taiwan, and Thailand have recovered organs from brain-dead patients (14). New programs and organ donation initiatives are also rapidly expanding in Latin America and the Baltic States (15,16).

Until recently, the United States has been unique with the actual use of transplant coordinators in the organ donation process. But many other countries such as Australia, the United Kingdom, and Canada are now recruiting coordinators, who offer the option of organ donation to families of potential organ donors (17). In addition, public and professional education programs and better administration of true organ donor potential are becoming more prevalent (18).

TABLE 10-1. *Establishment of transplant organizations around the world*

Years	Location
1967	EuroTransplant—Austria, Belgium, the Netherlands, Germany, Luxembourg
1968	France Transplant
1969	Scandiatransplant—Denmark, Finland, Iceland, Norway, Sweden
1972	United Kingdom Transplant Service—United Kingdom, Ireland
1975	Hong Kong
1985	Hellenic Transplant Service—Greece
1986	United Network for Organ Sharing—United States
1986	Singapore
1990	Organization National de Transplantes—Spain
1992	Taiwan
1994	Etablissement Francais des Greffes—Replaces France Transplant
1995	Balttransplant—Estonia, Lithuania, Latvia
1996	PRO-DONA—Mexico

IMPLICATIONS OF LEGISLATION

The Uniform Anatomical Gift Act of 1968 (see Chapter 8) legalized organ donation (19), but also specified who could give consent for organ donation and outlined what types of facilities could receive the organs and how the organs may be used. After the Uniform Determination of Death Act, the next major legislation was the 1984 National Organ Transplant Act (20). This act initiated federal oversight of organ donation and transplantation. Included in this act were provisions to provide grants for the planning, establishment, initial operation, and expansion of qualified OPOs, and ban the interstate sale of human organs. A Task Force on Organ Transplantation was also established under the auspices of this act to study policy issues involving organ donation and transplantation.

One Task Force recommendation was the establishment of policies requiring that the legal next-of-kin of every brain-dead potential organ donor be approached about organ donation, known as required request (21). This recommendation was carried out with the enactment of the Omnibus Budget Reconciliation Act of 1986 (22). Hospitals that receive Medicare or Medicaid funding are required to have policies to identify potential organ donors and assure that the legal next-of-kin of every potential organ donor is made aware of the option of organ and tissue donation and their option to decline. This act also required hospitals to comply with UNOS rules regarding the allocation of donated organs. While this act threatened to withhold federal Medicare and Medicaid funding if a hospital was non-compliant, no system was in place to determine compliance. Most states had also passed their own required request laws by 1988.

The most recent and substantial regulations passed since the Uniform Anatomical Gift Act are the Health Care Financing Administration's 42 CFR Part 482 rules enacted in 1998 (23). These regulations require that every death or imminent death in a hospital be reported to the OPO so that the OPO can determine medical suitability for organ, tissue, and eye donation. It also states that only OPO representatives or individuals who have been trained by the OPO are allowed to request consent for organ and tissue donation. Compliance with the regulations is to be monitored through medical record reviews performed by HCFA surveyors and regional offices. If a hospital is determined to be non-compliant, it may jeopardize its eligibility to participate in the Medicare and Medicaid program.

CRITERIA OF ORGAN DONATION

Potential organ donors and practices may vary nationwide within guidelines set by UNOS. Organs are routinely recovered from donors who are 2 days to 85 years old, but organ donors over the age of 50 account for 10–20% of all donors (1,24). Organs have been recovered from donors with prior cancer, hepatitis B and C, and many other diseases that would have been prior contraindications to organ donation. Cause of brain death generally does not impact organ donation; organs have been successfully recovered from donors whose cause of brain death was from trauma, intracranial hemorrhage, brain tumor (25), suicide and homicide, anoxia, poisoning (26), and even bacterial or viral meningitis (27). In the past, the stereotypical organ donor was

TABLE 10-2. *Primary diagnosis of transplant recipients by organ[a]*

Organ	Diagnosis
Heart	Coronary artery disease, cardiomyopathy, congenital heart disease
Lung	Emphysema/chronic obstructive pulmonary disease, cystic fibrosis, idiopathic pulmonary fibrosis, alpha-1-antitrypsin deficiency, primary pulmonary hypertension
Liver	Noncholestatic cirrhosis, cholestatic liver disease, acute hepatic necrosis, biliary atresia
Intestine	Short gut syndrome
Pancreas	Juvenile diabetes mellitus
Kidney	Glomerular diseases, diabetes mellitus, hypertension, autosomal dominant polycystic kidney disease

[a] UNOS Scientific Registry Data.

a young person declared brain dead following a motor vehicle accident. Today, less than half of the organ donors die from trauma.

Currently, organs that can be recovered for transplantation include the heart (28), lungs (29), liver (30), kidneys (31), pancreas (32), and small intestine (33). Recipients of organs require transplantation for a wide variety of diseases that cause end-stage organ failure. The primary diagnoses of organ transplant recipients are listed in Table 10-2. Tissues such as bone, heart valves, and eyes for corneal transplantation can also be recovered after the organ recovery. Donation of these tissues is not limited to brain-dead organ donors and with the consent of the next-of-kin may be recovered from any eligible patient after cardiac arrest.

ORGAN DONOR SHORTFALL

While the number of recipients on the UNOS waiting list has tripled in the last nine years, the number of organ donors has increased only approximately 30%. The United States statistics amassed by UNOS are shown in Figure 10-1. The waiting list as of December 1999 was 72,255 for all organs combined. The recipient deaths on the waiting list for the same year were 6,448. There are now more deaths of recipients waiting than there are organ donors per year. Estimates calculated through medical record reviews place the organ donation potential in the United States at 15,000 to 20,000 (3–5,34). As expected, the single largest factor inhibiting the number of organ donors is the consent rate. While several surveys, including the nationwide 1992 Gallup survey, place support for organ donation at about 90%, the national consent rate for organ donation remains below 50%. The Gallup survey also indicated only 52% of the respondents had discussed their wish to be an organ donor with family members in the event of brain death (2). If a family member had previously indicated a desire to be an organ donor, 93% of the respondents would be likely to honor their request (2).

While organ donor cards and driver's license check boxes for organ donation are useful, OPOs and transplant surgeons are reluctant to proceed with organ donation unless additional consent is obtained from the legal next-of-kin because the family can override any of these documents (36). Therefore, a signed organ donor card is not

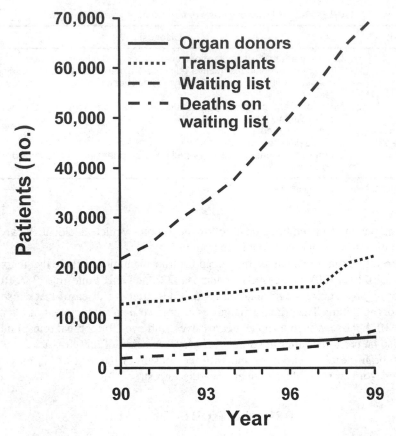

FIG. 10-1. Graphic representation of organ donors and needs. (From United Network of Organ Sharing, with permission.)

a legal document in most states and is only helpful to show the next-of-kin the patient's prior wishes with regard to organ donation.

Dispelling myths and misconceptions about organ donation should be part of an education program. Fictional books and television programs portray organ donation and transplantation inaccurately (36,37). Unfortunately, newscasts and documentaries have featured kidney stealing and black market organ trading. Transplantation in celebrities has been performed without evidence of preferential treatment although some concern exists. Mickey Mantle, a famous baseball player with hepatic cancer, received a transplant two days after being placed on the waiting list (compared with average 67 days waiting list). Unfortunately this raised questions about inappropriate consideration of urgency, but he survived his transplant for only a short time due to complications of cancer. More likely, his blood type and the severity of illness resulted in a rapid transplant. After his death, his family admirably established a foundation to promote organ and tissue donation ("Be a Hero, Be a Donor").

Another incident in the United Kingdom raised questions about inappropriate allocation of organs. In July 1998, the family of a brain-dead patient gave consent for organ donation with the condition the organs only go to white recipients. This wish was honored, but fortunately the organs were transplanted into recipients who would have received them without the condition mandated by the donor family (38).

While in the end, the U.K. case and Mickey Mantle's transplant did not deviate from accepted practice, there was a perception of impropriety by the media and the public. Transplant professionals must hold themselves to the highest ethical standards and confidentiality when allocating organs. Any forms of prejudice or selection cannot be tolerated in the current organization of organ allocation (38).

Education of health care professionals is needed in two main areas. First is aggressive identification of potential organ donors. One large study of 10,681 hospital deaths found that 13% of potential organ donors were either not identified or consent for organ donation was not requested from the next-of-kin (39). Second is clarification of the organ donation process. Following the reporting of potential organ donors to the OPO, communication of brain death to the family and cooperation with the OPO to request consent for organ donation should follow. Evanisko and associates (40) reported in 1998 that less than one third of 1,061 critical care nurses and physicians received training on explaining brain death and requesting organ donation to families. Similarly, McNamara and Beasley found only 25% received training on explaining brain death and grief counseling and 33% received training on the donation consent process (41). However, in some hospitals with high donation rates, less than 53% of the critical care staff received training. Moreover, the results of a European Donor Hospital Education Program, a 1-day workshop, indicated enhanced communication skills in physicians but not nursing staff. The effectiveness of this program on donation rates has not been studied (42).

REFERRAL AND REQUEST

All patients, regardless of age, past medical history, or current organ function, who have been declared brain dead or where brain death is imminent, should be referred to the hospital's designated OPO (23). Early referral but only when brain death is imminent allows the OPO coordinator an opportunity to determine medical suitability for organ donation (43,44).

The responsibility to determine medical suitability for organ donation should be relegated to the OPO. After review of the potential donor's medical history and current organ function on site or by phone, the OPO coordinator may determine (in conjunction with local transplant surgeons or the OPO medical director) whether the patient is a suitable candidate for organ donation. This determination is ultimately based on the probability of successfully transplanting at least one organ. Absolute contraindications to organ donation may include infectious diseases (notably HIV and hepatitis V), potentially transmissible malignancies (possibly including primary brain tumors manipulated by biopsy or ventriculostomy), and most commonly organ failure, which will result in primary non-function of the organ in the recipient (24). The final decision on suitability is often left to the discretion of the transplant surgeon.

After determination of suitability for organ donation, the OPO coordinator, attending physician, and ICU nurse should discuss the timeline of brain death testing, approach of the family for organ donation, care and support of the family, and medical management of the potential donor.

While the national estimated consent rate average is 45% to 50%, actual rates, as expected, vary substantially (3–5). There is some indication that the approach of family by a person not involved with discussion of brain death or a joint approach with the attending physician may result in 20% to 70% higher consent rates (41,45–52).

Gortmaker found, in addition, two modifiable factors: (a) donation requested in a quiet, private place (we have heard a physician yelling across the ICU "Oh yeah, what about donation") and (b) decoupling—i.e., the family understands and accepts brain death before discussion on organ donation is begun (49). DeJong et al. found in a survey of donor and non-donor families that 80% of donor families had a good understanding of brain death but a decrease to 50% in families who denied consent (45).

Communication of hopeless prognosis to the family is the first step in preparing a family for the diagnosis of brain death. The declaration of brain death should not come as a surprise to the family ("breaking bad news"), and with intermittent contacts, they should become aware of imminent death from a catastrophic brain injury. Rarely is the progression so quick that it completely overwhelms the physician and family. Ideally, families should be told that brain death testing may be performed, and that they will be informed when the clinical examination will start. Although one may argue that family observation of brain death testing may be helpful for those families who are having difficulty understanding the concept of brain death, there is no data that their actual presence will have a convincing effect. A clinching argument against the family present is that spinal reflexes may occur during the apnea test provocation. If spinal reflexes have been noted by family members, time must be taken to explain that the spinal cord and peripheral nerves are still functional and reflexes remain.

After brain death testing is complete, a meeting with all present family members should be arranged. However, before brain death and organ donation are discussed, the physician or OPO should have inquired about possible cultural or religious objections (see Chapters 7 and 8). The family should be told in unequivocal and non-technical terms that the patient is dead and not here anymore. Time should be allowed for grief, which may be of cataclysmic proportion in some family members, and others may direct anger toward the health care staff or even destroy furniture in the waiting room. Occasionally families dissolve into hysteria and collective grieving, which is characterized by shouting, crying, or fainting, significantly interfering with requests for donation. Many families recover quickly and regain a sense of realism. After this moment of grief, it may be necessary to repeat the inevitability of brain death. One may explain brain death as follows:

> The brain has stopped working entirely and activity, even a shred of function, cannot be brought back. No blood is flowing to the brain from very high pressure inside the brain due to swelling and therefore even the remaining cells have died. The heart will continue to pump as long as we push oxygen in the lungs using the ventilator and add drugs to keep a normal blood pressure. We would like you to see your loved one, but you will

not see an ashen gray person but someone who looks asleep. This makes it hard for everyone to understand this condition, but we are 100% certain the brain is dead. With our own ICU technology we can keep this lifeless body intact for days, even weeks, but it does not make sense . . . We are so sorry that this had to happen . . . We know that you are devastated . . . It is not fair . . . You will have a chance to say good-bye at anytime you are ready and we will be around here in the unit to comfort you. Is there anything we can get for you?

Understandably, families who have just lost a loved one are powerless, helpless, confused, and have short attention spans and their perception of events may be skewed (53). Organ donation is not mentioned at this time, but one may say,

There are some decisions that the family needs to make, after you have some time to spend together and paid your last wishes. We will be back to discuss some options.

Studies of the process of organ donation consent have shown that when the request for organ donation occurs simultaneously with the communication of brain death, the consent rate is 20-40% lower than if the request is separated from the explanation of brain death (46–48,51,52). Garrison et al. (52) reported that a temporal separation of the explanation of brain death before the request for organ donation yielded a donor success in 65% compared to a prior 18% consent rate when the discussion of death and donation were combined (49–52). Von Pohle found similar results with two- to threefold increase in consent rate in his study of 71 families approached for organ donation consent (46). Kay and Barone (51) reviewed 177 requests for organ donation over a one-year period. The consent rate for OPO coordinators approaching the family alone was substantially higher than a hospital staff member (47% vs. 4%).

Truly, organ donation should not be discussed with the family until their loved one is brain dead. However, as public education and experiences with organ donation and transplantation increase, more families approach physicians or nurses about their donation options, often before brain death is declared (54). We believe that if a family asks questions about donation, it is better to postpone this discussion and explain the present condition of the patient. However, when pressed by the family, time should be allowed to answer specific questions.

Once the family is ready for discussion of donation (time interval probably within 30 min after notification of brain death), the type of organs (kidney, heart, liver) and tissues that can be donated should be discussed (45–54). The benefits to the recipients should be specifically discussed and it is important for families to understand the high success rates for organ transplantation:

A wonderful gift of life for a person on a waiting list who otherwise will die within months . . . many lives can be saved by one person alone.

The consent will apply to all possible organs and this should be clarified.

Many families of potential organ donors have three concerns about organ donation: cost, timing, and disfigurement (45–55). The family should be assured the entire cost of the organ donation process is paid for by the OPO. Generally, this includes all costs from the time of brain death declaration and consent until the donor's care is transferred after the organ recovery to the medical examiner or funeral home. While the timing varies due to geographic location of the hospital and number of organs evaluated for transplant, the family should be given an approximated time for the entire process. On average it takes 12 h from the time of consent until the start of the recovery of organs in the operating room (56). The organ donation process should be explained in two parts, the evaluation and placement phase and "organ recovery" (harvesting is a disrespectful term) in the operating room. The family should understand all of the organs will be tested to determine suitability for transplantation, and testing may include blood tests, chest x-rays, echocardiograms, and coronary angiography. After the organs are evaluated they are matched with recipients on the waiting list. The family should be informed that the recovery process is done by trained transplant surgeons. A single incision is made from below the navel to just above the sternum. After the surgery the incision is closed and the donor is transferred to the medical examiner (if an autopsy is planned), or to the funeral home. The utmost respect and dignity are guaranteed. The family should be reassured that organ donation generally does not interfere with the type of funeral service (such as an open casket funeral). The family will receive a letter after the donation to tell them what organs could be transplanted and limited information about the recipients. A certificate of appreciation is sent as well (see Appendix). However, organ donation is an anonymous process and every effort is made to ensure the anonymity of both the donor and organ recipients.

The issue of correspondence and contact between donor families and recipients has been the subject of debate. While policies vary nationwide, anonymous correspondence between donor families and transplant recipients should be facilitated through the OPO. Contact with the recipients has been granted, when approved by the recipient, and some encounters have been very successful.

ORGAN DONOR PROCESS, EVALUATION, AND ALLOCATION OF ORGANS

A general overview of the donation process from the time of brain death declaration until care of the organ donor is transferred to the funeral home is shown in Figure 10-2.

For cases that fall under the local medical examiner's jurisdiction, permission to proceed with organ donation must be secured either before consent is requested from the family or immediately thereafter. One retrospective study found medical examiners refused to grant permission in one of 10 medical cases in 1992 that fell under their jurisdiction and the authors speculated that approximately 3,000 people may have been denied a transplant in a two-year study period (57). While there have been no reported cases where a criminal investigation or prosecution was impeded by organ donation, OPOs have developed strategies to enhance relationships with medical examiners, secure permission to proceed with organ donation, and increase the number of organs available for transplantation.

Shafer et al. (57) constructed the following guide after a 1993 survey of all OPOs: providing blood, urine, or other specimens for the medical examiner; inviting the medical examiner to attend the surgical recovery; obtaining additional examinations

Organ Donation Process

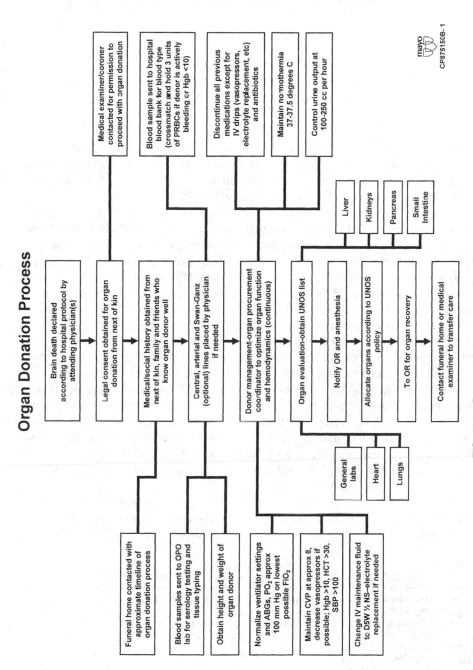

FIG. 10-2. Organ donation process flow diagram.

TABLE 10-3. *Serology tests for all organ donors*

HIV I and II
HTLV I and II
HCV
HBsAg
anti-HBc
CMV
RPR/STS
HBs/Ab, HIV p24 antigen (EBV optional)

for the medical examiner such as CT scans, MRI, echocardiogram, and other diagnostic and laboratory tests; videotaping the organ recovery; and providing follow-up on the condition of the organs recovered and status of the recipients after transplant. These recommendations, however, have not been validated.

After obtaining consent from the family and medical examiner, a detailed medical and social history should be obtained from the family. A positive HIV test disqualifies a donor but an accurate social history for homosexual relations, intravenous drug abuse, or incarceration that are at high risk for exposure to infectious diseases is obligatory (56). Nonetheless, incidental cases have been reported of HIV transmission from donor to recipients despite a negative HIV test at the time of donation (58). The history may identify prospective donors who are in the window period (24 to 28 days) from time of infection until the antigen or antibody can be detected by serological testing (59).

A blood sample should be sent to the hospital laboratory for immediate type and crossmatch because it may take up to 6 h when the laboratory is geographically distant. One study found a failure to determine blood type at the start of the donor management phase delayed the organ recovery for nearly 2 h (60). Blood (or tissue) samples are subsequently sent to an OPO-directed designated lab for serological testing (Table 10-3) and tissue typing. While the organ recovery may begin without the results, serological testing must be completed prior to transplantation of the organs (61). Tissue typing or identification of the Human Lymphocyte Antigens (HLA) is less critical than the serological testing, however, the results are critical to the allocation of kidneys and pancreas (62,63).

Organ evaluation should proceed with laboratory tests outlined in Table 10-4. Prior to diagnostic testing of the heart and lungs, attempts should be made to achieve hemodynamic stability. Often at the start of the donor management phase, the donor

TABLE 10-4. *Laboratory tests used in evaluation of multi-organ donor*

General (obligatory for all organ donors)—electrolytes (Na, K, Cl, CO_2), BUN, creatinine, glucose, CBC, calcium, magnesium, phosphorus, blood cultures (two sets from separate sites) (not from arterial or central venous lines), DIC panel (if DIC is suspected)
Liver—AST, ALT, total and direct bilirubin, GGT, alkaline phosphatase, LDH, PT, and PTT
Kidneys—urinalysis, urine culture
Heart—CPK with MB band, troponin
Pancreas—amylase, lipase
Lungs—arterial blood gases, sputum, Gram stain

TABLE 10-5. *Heart and lung donor evaluation*

Heart
  12-lead ECG
  Echocardiogram (transesophageal route preferred)
  Coronary angiography (for organ donors >40 years of age or those with cardiac risk factors
    such as hypercholesteremia, obesity, diabetes, or convincing family history of heart dis-
    ease)
  Swan-Ganz readings (optional)
  Cardiology consult
Lung
  Chest x-ray
  Arterial blood gas
  PEEP
  Bronchoscopy
  Oxygen challenge test
  Pulmonary consult

volume status is decreased as a result of diuresis from diabetes insipidus or administration of osmotic agents to reduce intracranial pressure. Efforts should be made to
gradually replace fluids but also to reduce vasopressor agents prior to obtaining the
echocardiogram. Results of an echocardiogram obtained during hemodynamic instability may be skewed due to hypovolemia and inotropic drugs. Evaluation of the heart
and lungs is outlined in Table 10-5. Once laboratory and diagnostic test data are
available, organ allocation can proceed according to current UNOS policy (63). Organ allocation policy changes frequently, and involved parties should contact UNOS
website for updated policies (www.unos.org). Anesthesia and operating room (OR)
personnel should be contacted well in advance of the organ recovery start time to allow for preparation of personnel and equipment.

Personnel required in the operating room for the organ recovery include: nursing
staff, an anesthesiologist, transplant surgeons, OPO coordinators, and organ preser-
vationists (64–67). Generally, multiple transplant teams will participate in the organ
recovery. One transplant team per thoracic organ and one team for all of the abdominal organs usually participate in the recovery. After the organ recovery is complete,
the body is transferred to the medical examiner or funeral home.

MEDICAL MANAGEMENT OF THE BRAIN-DEAD ORGAN DONOR

Brain death affects nearly every organ system (see Chapter 2). Complications of
brain death that may impact the organ donation process include: hypotension, diabetes insipidus, hypothermia, electrolyte abnormalities, coagulopathy, anemia, hypoxia, cardiac arrhythmia, and arrest (66–72). Medical management of the donor is
aimed at anticipating the normal physiologic sequelae of brain death and achieving
optimal organ perfusion and cellular oxygenation, minimizing ischemic injury. Following the declaration of brain death, care of the donor shifts to optimizing organ perfusion and protection. The initial medical management of the brain injured patient in
conjunction with cerebral resuscitation with osmotic diuresis, fluid restriction and
hyperventilation may compound many of the pathophysiologic outcomes of brain

death. Hypotension initially due to vasoparesis is worsened by untreated diabetes insipidus or diuretic-induced hypovolemia, hypothermia and electrolyte disorders (73–75). Despite maximum physiologic support, cardiac arrest occurs in 80% of adults within 48 to 72 h of brain death (see Chapter 2). We have developed an adult donor management protocol that provides a comprehensive guide for the clinician, critical care nursing staff, and organ procurement coordinator managing the brain-dead organ donor and can be found in the Appendix to this chapter.

Optimizing Oxygenation

Pulmonary edema and hypoxemia are due to central, cardiac, or intrinsic pulmonary causes (76–78). Goals of ventilatory management should include maintenance of a Pao_2 greater than 100 mm Hg with the lowest possible FIo_2 setting, and aimed at a normal pH (7.35 to 7.45) and $Paco_2$ (35 to 45 mm Hg) (76,78). Ventilator modes, commonly set to attain hypocarbia, should now be adjusted to include tidal volume of 10 to 12 cc/kg, positive end-expiratory pressure (PEEP) of 5 cm H_2O, and a respiratory rate that produces a $Paco_2$ of 35 to 45 mm Hg. While respiratory acidosis and alkalosis are corrected by changes in minute ventilation, metabolic acidosis as indicated by a negative base deficit requires treatment with sodium bicarbonate to improve in tissue perfusion. Frequent arterial blood gas measurements with appropriate ventilatory adjustments and good pulmonary toilet at least every 2 h using aseptic technique are essential (77–80). If sudden hypoxemia occurs as indicated by an Spo_2 < 95%, the endotracheal tube and ventilator should be checked to ensure proper positioning and function. The inspired concentration of oxygen and minute volume should be adjusted, with verification of the Pao_2 at greater than or equal to 100 mm Hg. Levels of PEEP in excess of 7.5 cm H_2O and peak inspiratory pressure greater than 30 cm H_2O are best avoided because of the detrimental effects on venous return to the heart, cardiac output, regional blood flow and possible barotrauma with lung injury. A chest radiograph should be obtained to rule out pneumothorax and determine the presence of infiltrates, atelectasis, or edema. Acute pulmonary edema in normotensive donors may respond to treatment with the application of PEEP in combination with diuretics, nitroglycerin and morphine (81). Central hemodynamic monitoring with a pulmonary artery catheter may be useful before treatment is initiated. Bronchodilator therapy may be efficacious when bronchospasm is suspected (72).

In the face of worsening hypoxemia, coagulopathy, profound hypothermia or refractory hypotension, the organ recovery surgery should proceed immediately to prevent ischemic injury to transplantable organs. The FIo_2 should be increased to 100% for transport to the operating room. The important exception is during heart-lung retrieval, when an FIo_2 less than 40% is desirable to minimize the possible effects of oxygen toxicity and atelectasis to the lungs.

Maintaining Hemodynamic Stability

As alluded in Chapter 2, brain-stem injury produces a sequence of hemodynamic events evolving from a massive catecholamine surge with hypertension and tachycardia to hypotension caused by a decrease in systemic vascular resistance and hypovolemia. Factors contributing to this hemodynamic instability include hypothermia, electrolyte disorders, myocardial dysfunction, and possible endocrine abnormalities. Initial therapy should be directed toward aggressive restoration and maintenance of the intravascular volume and the temporary use of vasoactive drugs, as needed. The specific organs to be retrieved determine type of fluid management, ideal central venous pressure (CVP) and the choice of allowable maximum doses for pressor support.

Targeted hemodynamic goals are described as the "rule of 100's" (73). This includes maintaining a minimum systolic blood pressure of 90 to 100 mm Hg (mean arterial pressure of 65 mm Hg), CVP $<$ 10 mm Hg, pulmonary capillary wedge pressure, PCWP $<$ 10 mm Hg, systemic vascular resistance (SVR) $<$ 1000 dynes/s^5, and heart rate $<$ 100 beats/min with a urine output $>$ 100 cc/h.

Treatment of hypovolemia causing hypotension, as indicated by a CVP $<$ 6 mm Hg, is initiated with fluid boluses of 5% albumin (82,83). The choice of crystalloid- or colloid-containing solution usually depends on institutional preference and the sensitivity of the liver and lungs to low osmotic pressure-mediated tissue edema. When only the kidneys are removed, the donor can be maximally fluid-loaded; otherwise, overhydration may precipitate cardiac failure, pulmonary failure, or congestion of the liver causing ischemic cellular injury during cold storage. For lung or heart-lung retrieval, infusion of colloid is recommended, with limited use of crystalloid and early initiation of inotropic support to maintain a systolic blood pressure above 85 mm Hg and CVP between 6 and 8 mm Hg. With persistent hypotension despite volume replacement, vasopressor therapy should be initiated. Ideally these pressor drugs will be used in limited doses and discontinued before organ retrieval. Dopamine is the preferred drug of choice because at infusion rates of 2 to 10 μg/kg/min the glomerular filtration rate is increased as well as cardiac output while dilating the renal, mesenteric and coronary vasculature. An infusion of phenylephrine, epinephrine and norepinephrine may be useful to increase peripheral vascular tone, but they have the inherent risk of causing marked peripheral vasoconstriction or an increase in pulmonary artery pressure. Low-dose dopamine (2 to 4 μg/kg/min) may be used in conjunction for protective renal vasodilation. Dobutamine in combination with dopamine should be used where cardiac output is decreased due to reduced myocardial contractility.

It has been proposed in order to offset the natural course of metabolic deterioration in the donor and to improve cardiac and renal functional stability in the recipient to administer thyroid hormones. Although controversial (see Chapter 2), more than 50% of transplant groups administer thyroid hormones to hemodynamically "rescue" unstable donors who give evidence of anaerobic metabolism or profound hypotension refractory to volume resuscitation and therapy with multiple vasopressors (84–91). Physiologic resuscitation of the donor with hormonal replacement therapy may also include administering steroids, insulin with glucose and arginine vasopressin (84–90). However, increase in the number of organs for transplantation through thyroid hormone therapy has not been consistently documented (see Chapter 2).

Hypotension resulting from blood loss is treated with transfusion of packed erythrocytes to a target hematocrit of 30%, and 4 units should be readily available. Disseminated intravascular coagulation (DIC) is evident in up to 90% of patients with lethal head injuries. Correction of the prolongation in PT and PTT (vitamin K and fresh frozen plasma), thrombocytopenia (platelets) and decreased fibrinogen (cryoprecipitate) can be exceedingly difficult and may necessitate immediate organ retrieval due to uncontrollable bleeding (91,92).

Despite aggressive therapeutic efforts, all brain-dead patients eventually undergo terminal arrhythmias. When cardiac arrest ensues, immediate resuscitation should proceed according to standard cardiopulmonary resuscitation and advanced life support protocols, with the exception that bradycardia or asystole should be treated with rewarming and isoproterenol or epinephrine, as atropine is not effective in the brain-dead patient (93). Prolonged hypotension or cardiac arrest accounts for an estimated 15% to 20% of organ procurement operations in adult donors that are abandoned each year.

Maintaining Normothermia

Hypothermia is common in organ donors due to loss of thermoregulatory function, exposure to a cold ambient temperature and massive infusions of cold intravenous fluids or blood products. The consequences of hypothermia which are clinically significant include arrhythmias, myocardial depression, hypotension, hypoxia, diuresis, hyperglycemia and coagulopathy (94). Therapeutic intervention to maintain a core temperature above 36°C should be early and aggressive. Such interventions include the use of a circulating air warming blanket (95), fluid warmers, heated ventilator circuits and increasing the ambient temperature of the operating room.

Management of Diabetes Insipidus

Clinical evidence of diabetes insipidus occurs in the vast majority of brain-dead donors. A frequently massive urine output that bears no relationship to the intravascular fluid volume with worsening hypernatremia in conjunction with a low urinary sodium and osmolality is strongly suggestive of diabetes insipidus (see Chapter 2). Therapeutic intervention includes replacement of urinary losses with warmed iso- or hypotonic crystalloid solutions on a volume-for-volume basis plus 1 cc/kg/h, electrolyte supplements and the administration of antidiuretic agents when the urine output exceeds 200 cc/h or 3 cc/kg/h (96–98). Serum electrolyte and osmolality measurements should be made every 2 to 4 h. A controlled intravenous low-dose infusion of aqueous vasopressin (AVP), starting at 3 units/h, or bolus doses of desmopressin acetate (DDAVP), 0.3-μg initial dose followed by a total dosage of 10 to 40 μg over 24 h, administered at 6- to 8-h intervals, may be efficacious in increasing water and sodium reabsorption from the distal tubule and titrating the hourly urine output to 2 to 3 cc/kg. It is desirable to discontinue the

AVP infusion at least 1 h before surgical recovery of organs due to its dose dependent effect of generalized systemic vasoconstriction. When refractory hypotension is a problem vasopressin should be considered as second-line pressor therapy in combination with dopamine. Desmopressin may be the preferred agent due to its enhanced antidiuretic potency, virtual absence of vasopressor and oxytocic activity and a prolonged half-life and duration of action compared with AVP (96–98).

Maintaining Glucose Homeostasis and Electrolyte Balance

Hyperglycemia may result from infusion of large volumes of glucose-containing solutions, peripheral insulin resistance resulting from the hormonal stress response, steroid administration and inotropic infusions. The major consequences of hyperglycemia include osmotic diuresis, an increase in plasma osmolality, ketosis and potential pancreatic graft dysfunction in the recipient following transplantation (99–101). Serum glucose, potassium and ketones must be monitored, and a sliding scale or continuous infusion of regular insulin (bolus 0.1 U/kg, followed by 0.5 to 2 U/h) is used to maintain the serum glucose level between 150 and 250 mg/dL. Electrolytes should be monitored every 2 h, because hypernatremia, hypokalemia, hypocalcemia and hypomagnesemia are common when aggressive fluid resuscitation is used. Correction of hypernatremia is critical as sodium levels in excess of 155 meq/dL may lead to a high incidence of graft loss after liver transplantation (99). Hypotonic solutions containing glucose are necessary for treating hypernatremic conditions but should be used with caution due to the potential for exacerbating hyperglycemia. A total of 20 mmol of potassium should be added to each liter of intravenous solution, with additional supplements as required to maintain the serum potassium level above 4 meq/L. Calcium chloride should be given for serum ionized calcium levels below 1.2 mmol/L. Hypomagnesemia can precipitate hypokalemia, hypocalcemia and cardiac arrhythmias and should be replaced with 4 grams of magnesium sulphate administered over 1 h. Hypophosphatemia often occurs as a physiologic consequence of brain death and may lead to rhabdomyolysis, hemolysis, platelet dysfunction and metabolic acidosis. Replacement with intravenous potassium phosphate or Nutraphos (two packets) via the nasogastric tube are both effective treatments.

Intraoperative Management of the Donor

The management is summarized in Table 10-6. Preoperative donor evaluation includes determining hemodynamic stability and pressor support, electrolytes and therapy for diabetes insipidus, oxygenation and pulmonary and renal function, coagulopathy and the degree of hypothermia. Routine anesthetic monitoring is supplemented with intra-arterial blood pressure, CVP and urine output with arterial blood gases, hematocrit, serum electrolytes and glucose measured every hour. Pancuronium will facilitate surgical exposure and avoid reflex muscular contractions.

TABLE 10-6. *Intraoperative management*

Low-dose isoflurane at beginning of incision
Neuromuscular junction blocker (pancuronium)
Discontinue medications except vasopressors and antibiotics
Fluid replacement: crystalloid, colloid, CMV-negative blood products
Fluid maintenance: total cc = urine output over preceding hour plus 1 cc/kg

Full anesthesia has been advocated by some (102); others use a small dose of isoflurane at the time of the incision to mute the sympathetic response. Pharmacologic interventions to improve organ preservation include: heparin (350 U/kg), diuretics, alpha-antagonists (chlorpromazine, phentolamine), PGE_1, and T3 or T4. Anesthetic support is necessary until aortic cross-clamping and start of *in situ* flushing of organs, after which all monitoring and supportive measures must be discontinued.

CONCLUSION

The diagnosis of brain death enables organ donation, and physicians have an obligation to address these matters. There is an increasing gap between demand and available organ supply. No condition should be attached to a donation and organs and tissue should be given altruistically.

Discussion with the family of the path to donation should be articulated in full because the shortage of organs is immense and demands immediate action. Alternative options for increasing organ donation are critically readdressing the overall donor criteria, expanding supply of living donors, split grafting or xenotransplantation (103).

APPENDIX

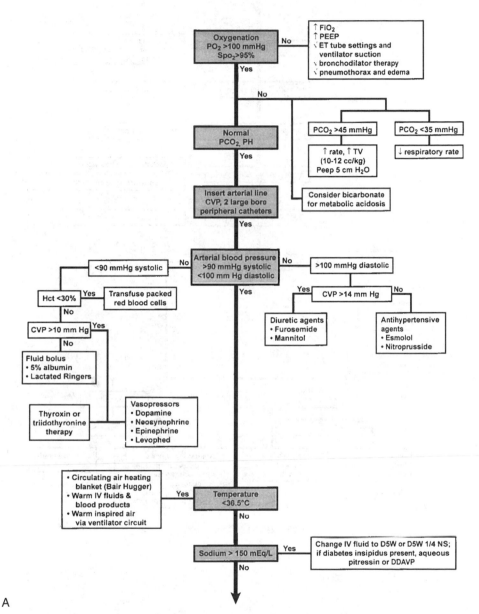

FIG. APP-1. Management and Procurement of the Organ Donor. PEEP, positive end expiratory pressure; CVP, central venous pressure; TV, tidal volume; HCT, hematocrit; IV, intravenous; K, potassium; Mg, magnesium; FFP, fresh frozen plasma; PT, prothrombin time; FSP, fibrogen split products; NG, nasogastric tube; HR, hour. *(continued)*

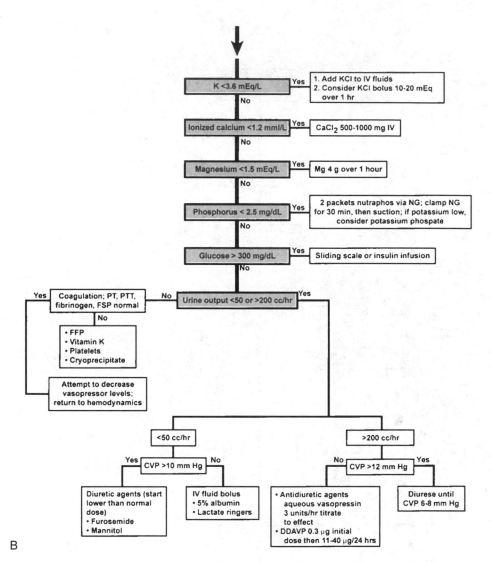

FIG. APP-1. *Continued.*

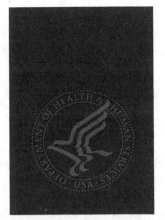

SURGEON GENERAL'S

Certificate of Appreciation

This certificate is presented
in honor of

_____

who gave the "Gift of Life"
to others.

U.S. DEPARTMENT OF HEALTH & HUMAN SERVICES
PUBLIC HEALTH SERVICE

David Satcher, M.D., Ph.D.
Assistant Secretary for Health
and Surgeon General

_____

Date

FIG. APP-2. Surgeon General Certificate of Appreciation.

REFERENCES

1. *1999 annual report of the U.S. Scientific Registry for Transplant Recipients and the Organ Procurement and Transplantation Network.* Rockville, MD: U.S. Department of Health and Human Services, Health Resources and Services Administration, Office of Special Programs, Division of Transplantation/Richmond, VA: United Network of Organ Sharing, 1999.
2. Gallup Organization. *The American public's attitudes toward organ donation and transplantation.* Boston: Partnership for Organ Donation, 1993.
3. Gortmaker SL, Beasley CL, Grenvik A, et al. Organ donor potential and performance: size and nature of the organ donor shortfall. *Crit Care Med* 1996;24:432.
4. Siminoff LA, Arnold RM, Caplan AL, et al. Public policy governing organ and tissue procurement in the United States. *Ann Intern Med* 1995;123:10.
5. Christiansen CL, Gortmaker SL, Williams JM, et al. A method for estimating solid organ donor potential by organ procurement region. *Am J Public Health* 1998;88:1645–1650.
6. Howard RJ. How can we increase the number of organ and tissue donors? *J Am Coll Surg* 1999; 188:317–327.
7. Beasley CL. Maximizing donation. *Transplant Rev* 1999;13:31–39.
8. McDonald JC. The National Organ Procurement and Transplantation Network. *JAMA* 1988; 259:725–726.
9. Pierce GA, McDonald JC. UNOS history. In: Phillips MG, ed. *Organ procurement, preservation, and distribution in transplantation,* 2nd ed. Richmond, VA: United Network of Organ Sharing (UNOS), 1996:2–5.
10. Department of Health and Human Services, Health Care Financing Administration. Medicare and Medicaid programs: conditions of coverage for organ procurement organizations. Final rule with comment. 42 CFR Parts 405, 482, and 485. *Federal Register* 1994;59:46500–46517.
11. Morphew-Magie C, Smith AB. The role of the recovery services coordinator. In: Klintmalm GB, Levy MF, eds. *Organ procurement and preservation.* Austin, Texas: Landes Bioscience, 1999:147–158.
12. Dutton SB. Certification of transplant coordinators by the American Board of Transplant Coordinators. *J Transplant Coord* 1996;6:210–214.
13. Bosch X. Spain leads world in organ donation and transplantation. *JAMA* 1999;282:17–18.
14. Takagi H. Organ transplantations in Japan and Asian countries. *Transplant Proc* 1997; 29:3199–3202.
15. Soberanes A, Vicente A, Nunez S, et al. New donation program at a Mexican social security institution: a Mexican model of cadaver donation and organ sharing—initial experience. *Transplant Proc* 1997;29:3307–3308.
16. Rosental R, Dainis B, Dmitriev P. BaltTransplant: a new organization for transplantation in the Baltic States. *Transplant Proc* 1997;29:3218–3219.
17. Schutt GR. Models for transplant coordination. *Transplant Proc* 1998;30:756–758.
18. Venturoli N, Venturi S, Taddei S, et al. Organ donation and transplantation as health programs in Italy. *Prog Transplant* 2000;10:60–64.
19. *Uniform Anatomical Gift Act.* 23 Bus L 919. 1968.
20. *National Organ Transplant Act.* Pub L No. 98-507, 3 USC g 301.
21. *Organ transplantation: issues and recommendations. Report of the Task Force on Organ Transplantation.* Rockville, MD: U.S. Department of Health and Human Services, Health Resources and Services Administration, Office of Organ Transplantation, 1986.
22. *Omnibus Reconciliation Act of 1986.* 42 USC 1320b-8.
23. *Medicare and Medicaid Programs; Hospital Conditions of Participation; Identification of Potential Organ, Tissue, and Eye Donors and Transplant Hospitals' Provision of Transplant Related Data.* 42 CFR Part 482.
24. Kauffman HM, Bennett LE, McBride MA, et al. The expanded donor. *Transplant Rev* 1997; 11:165–190.
25. Lewis DD, Vidovich RR. Factors influencing organ placement efforts in donors with brain tumors. *J Transplant Coord* 1996;6:37–38.
26. O'Connor KJ, Delmonico FL. Organ donation and transplantation from poisoned donors. *Transplant Rev* 1999;13:52–54.
27. McDowell JH, Zingaro BL. Organ recovery from a donor with presumed viral encephalitis: a case report and review. *J Transplant Coord* 1998;8:199–204.
28. Rodeheffer RJ, McGregor CGA. The development of cardiac transplantation. *Mayo Clin Proc* 1992; 67:480–484.

29. Benfield JR, Wain JC. The history of lung transplantation. *Chest Surg Clin North Am* 2000; 10:189–199.
30. Starzl TE. Liver transplantation. *Gastroenterology* 1997;112:288–291.
31. Brower PA, Harrison JH, Landes RR. Renal transplantation: history. *Urology* 1977;10:5–10.
32. Sutherland DE, Gruessner AC, Gruessner RW. Pancreas transplantation: a review. *Transplant Proc* 1998;30:1940–1943.
33. Margreiter R. The history of intestinal transplantation. *Transplant Rev* 1997;11:9–21.
34. Evans RW, Orians CE, Ascher NL. The potential supply of organ donors. *JAMA* 1992;267:239–246.
35. Lange SS. Psychosocial, legal, ethical, and cultural aspects of organ donation and transplantation. *Crit Care Nurs Clin North Am* 1992;4:25–42.
36. Hoskins S, Townley R. *Twisted lights.* Prairie Village, KS: Integrity Press, 1997.
37. Gerritsen T. *Harvest.* New York: Pocket Books, 1997.
38. Altruism and confidentiality in organ donation. *Lancet* 2000;355:765.
39. Siminoff LA, Arnold RM, Caplan AL. Asking for altruism when death occurs: who asks for organ donation and why? *Transplant Proc* 1996;28:3632–3638.
40. Evanisko MJ, Beasley CL, Brigham LE, et al. Readiness of critical care physicians and nurses to handle requests for organ donation. *Am J Crit Care* 1998;7:4–12.
41. McNamara P, Beasley CL. In: Cecka JM, Terasaki P, eds. *Clinical Transplants 1997.* Los Angeles: UCLA Tissue Typing Laboratory, 1997:219–229.
42. Morton J, Blok GA, Reid C, et al. The European Donor Hospital Education Programme (EDHEP): Enhancing Communication Skills With Bereaved Relatives. *Anaesth Intensive Care* 2000; 28:184–190.
43. Chabalewski F, Norris MKG. The gift of life: talking to families about organ and tissue donation. *Am J Nurs* 1994;94:28–33.
44. Rudy LA, Leshman D, Kay NA, et al. Obtaining consent for organ donation: the role of the health-care profession. *J S C Med Assoc* 1991;87:307–310.
45. DeJong W, Franz HG, Wolfe SM, et al. Requesting organ donation: an interview study of donor and nondonor families. *Am J Crit Care* 1998;7:13–23.
46. von Pohle WR. Obtaining organ donation: who should ask? *Heart Lung* 1996;25:304–309.
47. Niles PA, Mattice BJ. The timing factor in the consent process. *J Transplant Coord* 1996;6:84–87.
48. Franz HG, DeJong W, Wolfe SM, et al. Explaining brain death: a critical feature of the donation process. *J Transplant Coord* 1997;7:14–21.
49. Gortmaker SL, Beasley CL, Sheehy E, et al. Improving the request process to increase family consent for organ donation. *J Transplant Coord* 1998;8:210–217.
50. Klieger J, Nelson K, Davis R, et al. Analysis of factors influencing organ donation consent rates. *J Transplant Coord* 1994;4:132–134.
51. Kay NA, Barone BM. Optimizing the consent process for organ donation. *J S C Med Assoc* 1998; 94:69–75.
52. Garrison RN, Bentley FR, Raque GH, et al. There is an answer to the shortage of organ donors. *Gynecol Obstet Surg* 1991;173:391–396.
53. Coolican MB. Facing the sudden death of a loved one. *Crit Care Nurs Clin North Am* 1994; 6:607–612.
54. Verble M, Worth J. Adequate consent: its content in the donation discussion. *J Transplant Coord* 1998;8:99–104.
55. Pelletier M. The organ donor family members' perception of stressful situations during the organ donation experience. *J Adv Nurs* 1992;17:90–97.
56. Centers for Disease Control. Guidelines for preventing transmission of human immunodeficiency virus through transplantation of human tissue and organs. *MMWR* 43:1–17.
57. Shafer T, Schkade LL, Warner HE, et al. Impact of medical examiner/coroner practices on organ recovery in the United States. *JAMA* 1994;272:1607–1613.
58. Simonds RJ, Holmerg SD, Hurwitz RL, et al. Transmission of human immunodeficiency virus type 1 from a seronegative organ and tissue donor. *N Engl J Med* 1992;326:726–732.
59. Delmonico FL, Snydman DR. Organ donor screening for infectious diseases. *Transplantation* 1998; 65:603–610.
60. Emery S, Boysen L, Amberg B, et al. An analysis of time management related to the donation process. Presented at the Annual Meeting of the North American Transplant Coordinators Organization, New York, July 1998.
61. United Network of Organ Sharing (UNOS). *Policy 2.2.7.1.* Richmond, VA: UNOS, 1999.

62. Shroyer TW, Thomas JM. In: Phillips MG, ed. *Organ procurement, preservation, and distribution in transplantation*, 2nd ed. Richmond, VA: United Network of Organ Sharing, 1996, 207–220.

63. United Network of Organ Sharing (UNOS). *Policy 3.0*. Richmond, VA: UNOS, 1999.

64. Robertson KM, Cook DR. Perioperative management of the multiorgan donor. *Anesth Analg* 1990; 70:546–556.

65. Gelb AW, Robertson KM. Anaesthetic management of the brain dead for organ donation. *Can J Anaesth* 1990;37:806–812.

66. Scheinkestel CD, Tuxen DV, Cooper DJ, et al. Medical management of the (potential) organ donor. *Anaesth Intensive Care* 1995;23:51–59.

67. Nygaard CE, Townsend RN, Diamond DL. Organ donor management and organ outcome: a 6-year review from a level I trauma center. *J Trauma* 1990;30:728–732.

68. Kagiewska B, Pacholczyk M, Szostek M, et al. Hemodynamic and metabolic disturbances observed in brain-dead organ donors. *Transplant Proc* 1996;28:165–166.

69. Novitzky D. Detrimental effects of brain death on the potential organ donor. *Transplant Proc* 1997; 29:3770–3772.

70. Pratschke J, Wilhelm MJ, Kusaka M, et al. Brain death and its influence on donor organ quality and outcome after transplantation. *Transplantation* 1999;67:343–348.

71. Power BM, Van Heerden PV. The physiological changes associated with brain death—current concepts and implications for treatment of the brain dead organ donor. *Anaesth Intensive Care* 1995; 23:26–36.

72. Soifer BE, Gelb AW. The multiple organ donor: identification and management. *Ann Intern Med* 1989;110:814–823.

73. Boyd GL, Phillips MG, Henry ML. Cadaver donor management. In: Phillips MG, ed. *Organ procurement, preservation, and distribution in transplantation,* 2nd ed. Richmond, VA: United Network of Organ Sharing, 1996:81–93.

74. Holmquist M, Chabalewski F, Blount T, et al. A critical pathway: guiding care for organ donors. *Crit Care Nurse* 1999;19:84–98.

75. Emergency Cardiac Care Committee and Subcommittees, AHA. Guidelines for cardiopulmonary resuscitation and emergency cardiac care. Part III. Adult advanced cardiac life support. *JAMA* 1992; 268:2199–2241.

76. Fisher AJ, Dark JH, Corris PA. Improving donor lung evaluation: a new approach to increase organ supply for lung transplantation. *Thorax* 1998;53:818–820.

77. Sethman J, Kappel DF. Donor management strategies to maximize lung procurement. *J Transplant Coord* 1993;3:66–69.

78. McGiffin DC, Patterson GA, Zorn GL Jr. Donor lung procurement. In: Phillips MG, ed. *Organ procurement, preservation, and distribution in transplantation,* 2nd Ed. Richmond, VA: United Network of Organ Sharing, 1996:161–165.

79. Gluck E, Eubanks DH. Mechanical ventilation. In: Parrillo JE, Bone RC, eds. *Critical care medicine.* St. Louis: Mosby–Year Book, 1995:109–138.

80. Meyer DM, Wait MA, Jessen ME, et al. Optimal thoracic organ donor management. In: Klintmalm GB, Levy MF, eds. *Organ procurement and preservation.* Austin, Texas: Landes Bioscience, 1999:94–112.

81. Falk JL, O'Brien JF, Shesser R. Heart Failure. In: Rosen P, Barkin R, Danzl DF, et al., eds. *Rosen: Emergency medicine: concepts and clinical practice,* 4th ed. St. Louis: Mosby–Year Book, 1998:1645–1648.

82. Groeneveld ABJ, Thijs LG. Hypovolemic shock. In: Parrillo JE, Bone RC, eds. *Critical care medicine.* St. Louis: Mosby–Year Book, 1995:387–418.

83. Pennefather SH, Bullock RE, Dark JH. The effect of fluid therapy on alveolar arterial oxygen gradient in brain dead organ donors. *Transplantation* 1993;56:1418–1422.

84. Orlowski JP, Spees EK. The use of thyroxine (T-4) to promote hemodynamic stability in the vascular organ donor: a preliminary report on the Colorado experience. *J Transplant Coord* 1991;1:19–22.

85. Karayalcin K, Umana JP, Harrison JD, et al. Donor thyroid function does not affect outcome in orthotopic liver transplantation. *Transplantation* 1994;57:669–672.

86. McAdams DE, Bearden C, Headrick TR. Use of thyroid replacement therapy in donor management. *J Transplant Coord* 1995;5:117–120.

87. Mariot J, Sadoune LO, Jacob F, et al. Hormone levels, hemodynamics, and metabolism in brain dead organ donors. *Transplant Proc* 1995;27:793–794.

88. Cooper DKC, Basker M. Physiologic changes following brain death. *Transplant Proc* 1999; 31:1001–1002.

89. Novitzky D. Detrimental effects of brain death on the potential organ donor. *Transplant Proc* 1997; 29:3770–3772.
90. Novitzky D. Donor management: state of the art. *Transplant Proc* 1997;29:3773–3775.
91. Horne MK III. Hemorrhagic and thrombotic disorders. In: Parrillo JE, Bone RC, eds. *Critical care medicine.* St. Louis: Mosby–Year Book, 1995:1307–1321.
92. Kaufman HH, Hui KS, Kahan BD, et al. Clinicopathologic correlations of disseminated intravascular coagulation in patients with head injury. *Neurosurgery* 1984;15:34–42.
93. Vaghadia H. Atropine resistance in brain-dead organ donors. *Anesthesiology* 1986;65:711–712.
94. Farmer JC. Hypothermia and hyperthermia. In: Parrillo JE, Bone RC, eds. *Critical care medicine.* St. Louis: Mosby–Year Book 1995:1419–1428.
95. Sessler EL, Stoen R, Gosten B. The Bair Hugger[R] patient warmer significantly decreases heat loss to the environment. *Anesthesiology* 1989;71:A411.
96. Schrefer J, ed. Vasopressin. In: *Mosby's GenRx,* 9th ed. St. Louis: Mosby–Year Book, 1999.
97. Schrefer J, ed. Desmopressin acetate. In: *Mosby's GenRx,* 9th ed. St. Louis: Mosby–Year Book, 1999.
98. Pennefather SH, Bullock RE, Mantle D, et al. Use of low-dose arginine vasopressin to support brain-dead organ donors. *Transplantation* 1995;59:58–62.
99. Totsuka E, Dodson F, Urakami A, et al. Influence of high donor serum sodium levels on early postoperative graft function in human liver transplantation: effect of correction of donor hypernatremia. *Liver Transplant Surg* 1999;5:421–428.
100. Knochel JP. In: Isselbacher KJ, Braunwald E, Wilson JD, et al., eds. *Harrison's principles of internal medicine*, 13th Ed. New York: McGraw-Hill, 1994:2184–2193.
101. Gores PF, Gillingham KJ, Dunn DL, et al. Donor hyperglycemia as a minor risk factor and immunologic variables as major risk factors for pancreas allograft loss in a multivariate analysis of a single institution's experience. *Ann Surg* 1992;215:217–230.
102. Wace J, Kai M. Anesthesia for organ donation in the brain stem dead [Letter]. *Anesthesia* 2000; 55:590.
103. Gridelli B, Remuzzi G. Strategies for making more organs available for transplantation. *N Engl J Med* 2000;343:404–410.

Subject Index

Page numbers followed by f refer to figures; page numbers followed by t refer to tables.